Survival Skills for Nurses

Ruth Chambers

General Practitioner
Professor of Health Commissioning
Staffordshire University

Barbara Hawksley

Principal Lecturer
Community Nursing
Staffordshire University

Teeranlall Ramjopal

Associate Dean
School of Health
Staffordshire University

RADCLIFFE MEDICAL PRESS

©1999 Ruth Chambers, Barbara Hawksley, Teeranlall Ramjopal
Illustrations ©1999 Martin Davies

Radcliffe Medical Press Ltd
18 Marcham Road, Abingdon, Oxon OX14 1AA

British Library Cataloguing in Publication Data

A catalogue record for this book is available from the British Library.

ISBN 1 85775 339 9

Typeset by Advance Typesetting Ltd, Oxon
Printed and bound by Hobbs the Printers, Totton, Hampshire

CONTENTS

PREFACE

Nursing is no longer the job it once was. Nurses have progressed from a secondary role supporting doctors to relative autonomy and teamwork, and from performing basic care to specialised practice. In theory, these changes and many others resulting from the restructuring of the NHS should make the working conditions for nurses more satisfying. However, sometimes the excessive pressures from patients and managers, too few staff, inappropriate skill mix and poorly managed workplaces produce stress and demands that overshadow the rest of nurses' work. The focus on evidence-based practice illustrates the balance between change having the potential to increase job satisfaction, while at the same time being challenging and producing stress if sufficient help, support and time are not available to individual nurses to learn new skills.

Changes which are immense, swift and sometimes imposed from outside typically result in stress and turmoil for the individuals concerned. The three main components of stress are lack of control, lack of support and high demands, all of which are commonly encountered by staff working in today's NHS.

Survival is not only about learning to cope with the changed circumstances of nursing and the NHS, but also about how to flourish and enjoy one's working life. That is why this book takes you the reader on a path from becoming more aware of what is causing you stress at work and home, the effects of stress on you and how you usually react to it (Module 1), to looking at ways of enhancing your career and developing yourself further both as a person and as a professional (Module 6). The intervening sections, starting with Module 2, will increase your understanding of the range of options and solutions that are available to you to control stress or minimise it if you cannot obliterate it completely. In Modules 3 and 4 you are encouraged to practise being more assertive and to manage your time better, as these are two key skills which will help you to control your workload in a pro-active way and create more time for your own interests.

In Module 5, understanding more about what gives you job satisfaction and how you might increase it should help to make you more resilient to change. You need to develop survival skills that are integral to you, and that will help you to handle any significant stress or adverse life events that come your way. Your more highly developed personal and professional satisfaction should be a positive force that will protect you from disillusionment and low morale in years to come.

These six Modules make up the *Survival Skills* programme for nurses. They have evolved from the popular long-distance learning programme written as part of the Stress Fellowship of the Royal College of General Practitioners. A time allotment has been calculated for each Module to guide the reader as to how long it should take to read and reflect on the relevance of each Module for her or his situation, and to complete the exercises. You might work on your own, or alternatively seek a local tutor to provide feedback or organise a small group of nurses to undertake the *Survival Skills* programme together as part of clinical supervision, for example. Primary Care Groups or Trusts might encourage peer groups of nurses and other health care professionals to work through the programme in the same way. You might take your time and undertake one Module every few months, or you might complete them all one after another within a relatively short space of time. The beauty of a programme like this is that you can work at your own pace.

This *Survival Skills* programme should remind you of the many strengths and opportunities that you already have. Following the programme should build up your confidence in your own personal and professional qualities, so that by the end of the sixth Module you will agree that nursing is no longer the job it was – it is better!

Ruth Chambers
Barbara Hawksley
Teeranlall Ramjopal
July 1999

Ruth Chambers is a well known authority on the effects of stress at work on nurses and doctors. She has written and lectured extensively on the subject. **Barbara Hawksley** brings the community nursing perspective being a principal lecturer in community nursing and working closely with practice nurses, midwives, health visitors and other community nurses. **Teeranlall Ramjopal** has supervised the education of thousands of pre-registration nursing students. All three have witnessed the effects of stress on work colleagues of all levels of seniority in general practice and Trust settings, and helped many to overcome difficulties at work, and develop their nursing and medical careers.

Authors' Note

'**Workplace**' is the term that will be used throughout the course to denote the nurse's working environment, whether it is a general practice, hospital or community setting.

'**Nurse**' is the term that will be used throughout the course material to denote all types of nurse, including community nurses, specialist nurses and general nurses in NHS or private settings.

'**Community nurse**' is the term that will be used for a health visitor, practice nurse, district nurse, mental health nurse, learning disability nurse, occupational health nurse or any other nurse working in a community setting, e.g. a nursing home.

MODULE 1
Realising the causes and recognising the symptoms

AIMS

The aims of Module 1 are:

1 To help nurses to become more aware of the nature and causes of stress at work, and to learn to recognise it in themselves and others.

2 To help nurses to understand and appreciate the effects of stress on themselves and others.

3 To help nurses to realise the impact of adverse effects of stress on their work.

CONTENTS

The total time needed to work through the module will probably be about 10 hours, depending on the amount of time you spend reading and reflecting on how the information in the module applies to you before completing the exercises.

Below are the comments that some student nurses and nurse teachers made about stress.

Students

'There's so much to learn. It's all very new to me. I wonder if I'll be expected to know it all.'

'You're given so much information and I don't know whether I'll remember anything when I start on the ward.'

'Everybody seems to be under stress on the ward where I've just started. There are times when it's just you, a qualified nurse and a health care support worker, and you feel the pressure, and I constantly worry that I'll get it wrong. That's what stresses me.'

'To be honest with you the hard work doesn't stress me. I'm used to it being a mature student. I have two young children and believe you me there's nothing more stressful than having to cope, especially when they're ill. No, the work doesn't stress me, but the thought of getting it wrong, or doing things wrong does. I haven't seen a cardiac arrest yet. I'm dreading that. As I said, we're all under stress.'

'Community placements stressed me a lot. I haven't got my own transport and so I had to use the bus everywhere I was placed. I used to get worried about being late and people thinking I wasn't interested in community nursing. The other thing I found quite stressful is going into people's homes. You never knew how they'd react. Some were nice but for some of them, I wouldn't like to go on my own.'

Nurse teachers

'I get stressed when people expect so much from you and you just haven't got the time.'

'It seems that we've got to please so many bosses. We've got the Board (English National Board), the University, the Training Consortium, Regional Office (the National Health Service Management Executive Regional Office), the local Trusts (NHS Trusts), the clinical staff on the wards, not to mention the students themselves and the School – too many people to please, that's our problem.'

'There's not enough time to do what you want to do. And you know you can do most of what you're asked, if only they'd give you a bit more time. So you do things quickly and then you make mistakes and then you get it in the neck from someone up there and then you spend the rest of the week worrying about it.'

'Stress, what stress! I reckon you stress yourself. I don't get stressed that easily. I don't let things worry me, mate. I tell you, it's not worth it. Life is too short. I know I'm expected to do this and that. If I did everything people expect me to do at work, I tell you something, I'll not be here telling you about it, that's for certain. No, take it from me, it's not worth it. You've got to control things before they control you. That's my motto, for what it's worth.'

Below are some comments about sources of stress from one 'G'-grade Sister of a mixed medical and surgical ward:

- 'Shifts – internal rotation, swapping from nights to days or the other way round at short notice.'

- 'Demanding patients – particularly those who know they are paying; conflict with patients.'

- 'Consultants shouting.'

- 'General pressures – shortage of staff, expected to manage more with less.'

- 'Clinical pressures.'

- 'Knowledge-base stress – knowing that we don't know everything. Having to be on the ball on everything.'

- 'Having to keep to budget.'

Community nurses – some thoughts about stress

'Can't keep up with all the changes. You come to work one week, you're expected to do things one way and then a few weeks later you are told that it's not done that way any more. Sometimes I think changes are made just for the sake of it.' (Practice Nurse)

'Admin., admin. and more admin. – drives me mad.' (Health Visitor)

'Now that I'm attached to a practice, I seem to spend half my life travelling.' (District Nurse)

WHAT IS STRESS?

It's a word you hear almost every day. It is talked about in the newspapers, on the radio, at work and in people's homes. It is used so often that we should be able to define it clearly and precisely. However, that is not the case because stress can mean different things to different people. To a certain extent we would be justified in saying that stress is what people say it is, but this does not take us very far, particularly when dealing with stress is part of our professional role. As such there is an expectation that we should know more about stress than our clients or patients. Certainly one way of increasing our knowledge of the subject is to look at the various research findings or studies conducted on it.

The literature suggests that stress is very much about a person's perception of the pressure upon them. It is the product of a 'three-way relationship between demands on a person, that person's feelings about those demands and their ability to cope with those demands'.[1] So, putting yourself in this situation, a particular event or task can be very stressful for you on one day but not on another – all depending on how you are feeling and what other pressures are being exerted on you.

In general, stress occurs in situations where the workload is high, control over the workload is limited, and too little support or help is available. Many nurses and midwives would say that they know when they are feeling stressed even if they cannot specify exactly what stress is!

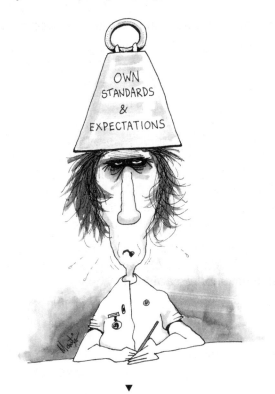

▼

What is stress?

Is stress bad for you? It depends on how much stress you are under, how long it is applied for, whether you feel powerless to stand up to the stress, or whether you can overcome it. There is a close relationship between your performance and demand. Low demand on an individual does not necessarily result in high performance.[2] On the contrary, a moderate amount of stress is necessary in order to perform well, not only at work but also in maintaining a zest for life. Therefore, on the one hand, absence of stress may lead to boredom, while on the other, too much stress over too long a period can render you indecisive, and leave you exhausted or 'burnt out'.

Are nurses 'special cases'? The average yearly absence for each nurse is 14 days – twice the national average.[3] It is said that in a typical week one million of the 24 million people in the UK's labour force took one day off work, and up to 40% of absenteeism in the workforce in general is thought to be due to mental or emotional problems. In 1994, for example, a newspaper article on 'white-collar' workers revealed that 'stress-related illness costs the nation 90 million days and £13 billion in absenteeism each year'.[4]

Over 360 000 working days are being lost each year in the NHS because of nurses' absence due to stress-related illness, according to a report by the secretary of the Royal College of Nursing in 1995.

Is stress an integral part of the job? If we accept that stress is a 'reflection of the wear and tear of life',[5,6] then nursing is not immune to it. But what is it about nursing that makes it so stressful?

In nursing and medicine, of course, caring for others creates additional stresses caused by daily exposure to human distress, ill health, death and dying. A study conducted in 1990 showed that dealing with death and dying was one of the greatest sources of stress for qualified as well as student nurses.[5] It could also be that part of the stress which nurses experience is related to the pressure generated by the image and expectations that the public has of nurses and other caring professionals. While it is understandable that mistakes at work can be very costly, the fear of getting things wrong can be a powerful source of stress.[6]

There is a strong link between demand – physical or psychological – and stress. Stress is related to the level of autonomy or control that a person has to meet such demand.[5] A study of nurse managers in the late 1980s revealed nine potential sources of stress.[7] These are:

1 workload[7–9]

2 working relationships with more senior colleagues

3 role conflict and ambiguity

4 dealing with death and bereavement[8–11]

5 the conflict between home and work

6 lack of career prospects

7 interpersonal relationships with patients/clients, relatives and colleagues[5,8,10]

8 lack of resources

9 keeping up with changes.[11]

(The additional references given in the lists above and below refer to other studies supporting these sources of stress.)

Another study based on 475 female nurse managers came up with a similar list.[12] In addition to the sources of stress listed above, other factors included the following:

• lack of confidence in carrying out certain procedures[5,9]

• having to carry out tasks in front of others[13]

• having to cope with ward-based practical assessments and course assignments.[8,14]

These last three points apply particularly to students in training or anyone who is working under the supervision of senior staff. They are also linked to keeping up with changes, which is another cause of stress. For example, students in training have to cope with changes in their placements so that, in a matter of weeks or months (probably not more than two or three) students move from one clinical setting to another. For instance, for 3 months a student may be on the children's ward, and they may then move to an adult ward, then on to a community placement, followed by a move on to nights, and then to a mental health placement, etc. On top of having to cope with differences in practice, not to mention the varying styles and expectations of the qualified nurses, students also have to pass the practical assessment, otherwise they fail to qualify. And all the while, like their qualified counterparts, they too find it very stressful to cope with the stresses that are intrinsic to the nursing job, such as death and bereavement.[15–17]

Other evidence also suggests that working in specialised settings such as the Special Care Baby Unit,[18–21] critical-care settings such as Intensive Care or a Coronary-Care Unit[22–26] or an Accident and Emergency department[27–29] can be more stressful than other areas of nursing practice.

However, it is important to bear in mind that stress is very much an individual matter. It is not the case that only those who work in such areas have legitimate claims to feel under stress. In reality, staff in all parts of the service can be affected. The trick, of course, is to learn to recognise it first in ourselves and then in other colleagues, so that we can do something about it.

Now consider your own work situation. Are you aware of when you are under stress and what is causing you to feel stressed? Are you aware when other colleagues are stressed? You may answer 'yes' on all counts. On the other hand, you may feel that because you are a nurse, you should manage other people's stresses but not your own. You might feel that you cannot admit to anyone that you are under stress or that you cannot cope. You think that to say so would be a sign of weakness, but this is not the case. The only way in which you are going to understand how stress is affecting you, and through you others around you at work and at home, is by identifying the sources, effects and consequent outcomes for *yourself*, discussing them with others at work and coming up with realistic solutions. You will not be able to solve your problems with stress in isolation from other people, just by reading books like this one and making resolutions that relate only to you.

The next section will start to look at the symptoms and effects of stress. Over time you should come to realise which of these are most applicable to you.

SYMPTOMS OF STRESS

Stress at work does not happen in a 'vacuum'. Pressures and problems at home often overflow into how someone feels and performs at work, and the effects of stress at work are often taken home and unfairly dumped there. Different people suffer various proportions and mixes of physical, mental, emotional and behavioural types of stress symptoms.

Stress can affect everyone. It often goes undetected or unacknowledged by the sufferers, who may have been warned by others to 'slow down', and have delighted in ignoring such advice and pushing themselves on regardless. It is often people with 'Type A' personalities who react in this way, and their particular characteristics will be explored a little later.

EXERCISE 1   Where are you now? What symptoms of stress are you suffering?

Look at the list below of behavioural and personal symptoms described by people suffering from stress at work. Tick the ones that you have experienced. When did you experience this – recently or in the past? Changes in feelings or behaviour may well indicate stress.

How many are significant symptoms of stress for you, or are they really quite trivial and unimportant? Circle the three most significant behavioural symptoms and the three most significant personal symptoms for you in the table below.

Behavioural symptoms	Tick the ones you have experienced	When did you experience this?
Shy away from paperwork Put things off Indecisive Shunt work away Work through all weekends Under-performing Less efficient Late for work Longer working hours but less done Breakdown in relationships Argumentative Irritable Accident prone Loss of interest in sex Overeating Withdrawal from relationships		
Personal symptoms	Tick the ones you have experienced	When did you experience this?
Feel anxious Palpitations Feel burdened Insomnia Panic/hyperventilation Reduced appetite Tired/drained Jumpy Difficulty in concentrating Depressed Nausea/indigestion Cynical Loss of confidence Lack of self-esteem Feelings of helplessness		

CAUSES OF STRESS

EXERCISE 2   Where are you now? Compare your causes of stress with those of others.

To find out whether these causes of stress apply to you, fill in the questionnaire below about what causes *you* stress at work. The causes of stress are not listed in any order of priority. Colleagues in the health service have identified them.[2] Tick whether these are sources of stress for you, ticking 'No stress', 'Somewhat stressful' or 'Very stressful' according to how significant you perceive that factor to be in causing you stress. At the same time, rank each factor from 1 to 10 according to how important a stress it is for you, where '1' is the most important source of stress for you and '10' is the least important.

Sources of stress	No stress	Somewhat stressful	Very stressful	Ranking
Not enough staff				
Too much work				
Working hours				
Feeling inadequately prepared to carry out certain clinical procedures				
Colleagues' attitudes				
Patient abuse or aggression				
Cardiac arrests				
Conflict with colleagues				
Patients' demands				
Complaints				
Dealing with death and bereaved relatives				
Lack of resources				
Study				
Assessments				
Demands made by doctors or managers				
Disorganised management at work				
Poor communication				
General ambience and comfort of workplace environment				
Other: (complete yours)				

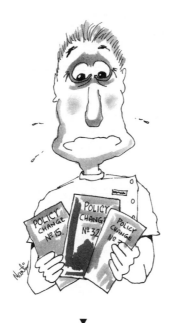

▼

Change and turmoil.

A study of qualified nurses, students and those who had left nursing came up with 26 potential sources of stress at work.[5] The tables below show the ranking of the top potential sources of stress identified by qualified nurses and students in order of impact on them, in relation to the factors listed in the previous questionnaire. If you are a qualified nurse who works in a hospital or the community, compare your response with the list in Table A. If you are a student nurse, then compare your response with the list in Table B.

Table A: Ranking of top five potential sources of stress reported by qualified staff

Sources of stress listed in questionnaire in Exercise 2	Trained nurses' ranking	Your ranking from Exercise 2
Not enough staff	1	
Conflict with colleagues	2	
Too much work	3	
Dealing with death and bereaved relatives	4	
Lack of resources	5	

Table B: Ranking of top nine sources of stress reported by student nurses

Sources of stress listed in questionnaire in Exercise 2	Student nurses' ranking	Your ranking from Exercise 2
Dealing with death and bereaved relatives	1	
Cardiac arrests	2	
Too much work	2	
Not enough staff	4	
Conflict with other colleagues	4	
Study and assessments	4	
Working hours	7	
Feeling inadequately prepared to carry out certain clinical procedures	8	
Patient abuse or aggression	9	

What is a Type A personality and what is its relationship with stress?

Since the 1950s, physicians and psychologists have been studying personality types.[30] Physicians in particular have looked at the connection between personality and the incidence of coronary heart disease. The results showed a tendency for there to be a high incidence of coronary heart disease among individuals who exhibited certain traits. These traits are collectively referred to as 'Type A'. This make-up in people's personalities also makes them more vulnerable to stress. They are thought to be highly demanding of themselves and others, driving themselves to be perfectionists. On the other hand, 'Type B' people are able to relax without feeling guilty, and to work without becoming agitated; they lack a sense of urgency, with its accompanying impatience, and are not easily roused to anger'.[31]

'Type A' behaviour is often learned in childhood, especially when the child strove to achieve in order to counteract his or her low self-esteem or self-worth. Although some professionals may believe that 'Type A' characteristics are a positive benefit in that they help them to get through their work quickly, in the longer term these characteristics are self-destructive. 'Type B' personalities can be just as successful and achieve just as much as 'Type A' personality types, at a slower but more steady pace. Because 'Type A' behaviour is often learned, it can be modified with practice.

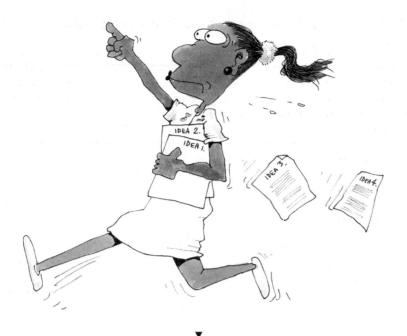

▼

Type A personality.

EXERCISE 3   Where are you now? Review your own personality type.

Please read through the list in Table A and tick those factors which you feel correspond to your own personality. Now rate how extreme you feel you are for each Type A characteristic listed below, out of a maximum score of 10. For example, if you think that your feelings are absolutely contained, then score '10' in that column. Alternatively, if you are very expressive of your feelings, then score '1'. Tick which factors you think encourage you to become over-stressed.

Table A

Type A characteristics	Rate factors that apply to you (score 1–10)	Tick which factors encourage stress in you
Highly competitive		
Hard driving		
Feelings contained		
Sets frequent deadlines		
Meticulous about details		
Does everything fast		

EXERCISE 3   Continued.

Table A *continued*

Type A characteristics	Rate factors that apply to you (score 1–10)	Tick which factors encourage stress in you
Ambitious		
Fidgety if kept waiting		
Intolerant of mistakes		
Does more than one task at a time		
Anticipates others in conversation		
Hard worker – few outside interests		
Feels angry/impatient in queues		
Feels responsible		
Aggressive		
High achiever		
Continual sense of time urgency		
Easily upset/angry over trivia		

Looking at the Table of Type A characteristic scores, pick the three highest scoring factors. Write down in Table B below which factors you have selected and what plan of action it might be possible to take in order to reduce each factor.

Table B

High-scoring Type A characteristic	Possible action
1	
2	
3	

EXERCISE 4   Where are you now? Complete a series of daily logs to check whether you have identified all your causes of stress comprehensively.

Make five photocopies of the unused form overleaf for monitoring stress at work. Fill in one each day for a typical week, recording any sources of stress and your usual reactions or responses (either good or bad). For example, 'bad' responses or behaviour might include snapping at a student after a row with the house officer, losing your temper inappropriately after a succession of interruptions to your work, or showing your irritation to a newly diabetic patient who did not follow your instructions. 'Good' responses or behaviour might include, for example, reorganising the ward's early morning routines, sharing your concerns with others, or making sure that you allowed more time to travel between your workbase and patients' homes.

These are just examples from different work settings – a ward or the community. It is important for you to consider *your personal working environment* and the activities that *you* view as being stressful for you.

Recording five days' worth of logs should ensure that you obtain a spread of busy and less pressured days. At the end of the week, review your recordings for all five days and write down your most common stressors at work and your usual responses on the summary log form which follows (on page 17).

Then repeat the exercise, completing stress logs for the time you spend outside work – at home or in other places or situations, during the weekend or before and after the working day. Photocopy three days' worth of stress log forms and, as before, record your usual responses to any stress outside work arising over the three days. Summarise the sources of stress arising outside the workplace and your usual responses on the summary log form. Stresses at home and in the environment may be inter-mingled with stresses at work, and it could be difficult to separate out exact causes and effects.

You could complete and monitor daily logs for activities and stress at work and outside work at the same time, but to do so might put you under too much pressure. If you are continually watching and analysing yourself all day long you may become fed up with this exercise and abandon it altogether.

Keep at it! If you want a break, stop doing the log for a day or two and start again later in the week, rather than stopping altogether.

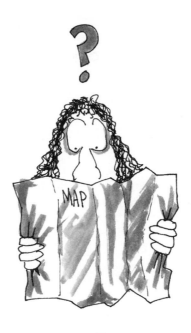

▼

Where are you now?

DAILY STRESS LOG AT WORK: Day and date: ....

Source of stress at work: My response:

....
....
....
....
....
....
....
....
....
....
....
....

Comments:

....

....

My overall stress level for today was: 0 1 2 3 4 5 6 7 8 9 10
(circle your reply)

DAILY STRESS LOG OUTSIDE WORK: Day and date: ....

Source of stress outside work: My response:

....

....

....

....

....

....

....

....

....

....

....

....

....

....

....

Comments:

....

....

My overall stress level for today was: 0 1 2 3 4 5 6 7 8 9 10
(circle your reply)

**SUMMARY STRESS LOG   Overview of sources of stress
and usual responses at work and outside work in week
beginning:** ....

Most frequent sources
of stress at work:

My usual response:

....

....

....

....

....

....

....

....

....

....

....

....

....

....

Most frequent sources
of stress outside work:

My usual response:

....

....

....

....

....

....

EFFECTS OF STRESS

The potential human and organisational costs resulting from the consequences of over-stressed staff are enormous. Improving the mental health of staff could increase the effectiveness of the whole organisation. Put simply, stress in nurses can affect more than just the quality of patient care. Relationships with other colleagues become more strained, the so-called 'working team' disintegrates, and the more people drift apart, the more pressure there is on individuals. Your competence is called into question, and before you realise it, stress has become a vicious cycle and you are caught in a downward spiral.

The list below summarises the known effects of stress on a workforce.[5,31]

Effects of stress in the workplace

- Reduced output
- Lack of creativity
- Increased errors
- Poor decision-making
- Job dissatisfaction
- Poor timekeeping
- Disloyalty
- Increased sick leave
- Increased complaints
- Premature retirement
- Absenteeism
- Accidents
- Thefts
- Organisational breakdown.

Translating these effects into the consequences of stress in nursing includes the following possibilities.

- When less is being achieved because staff are over-stressed, this also means that the workload builds up. This could result in staff refusing to work extra shifts to cope with the increased workload.

- An increased workload could also increase the likelihood of errors in, for example, the administration of drugs, or failure to attend to the needs of seriously ill patients.

- Not having the chance to reflect on your practice could also impede the opportunity to think creatively and improve the quality of patient care. Thus there is less likelihood of innovative practice developments, and fewer options of care are devised and offered to patients. Moreover, nurses who are stressed are more likely to resist changes and be unco-operative.

- Poor decision-making could result in a patient having a more prolonged stay in hospital. Alternatively, it could result in inappropriate action being taken, proving very costly for both the individual and the health service.

The effects of stress on individual nurses or other health care professionals are summarised under the following headings.

1 **Individual:** Symptoms could include changes in feelings, behaviour, thinking and general well-being, such as have been covered earlier in this module.

2 **Organisational:** Symptoms could include all aspects of performance at work, and relationships with others on other wards or departments or outside NHS bodies.

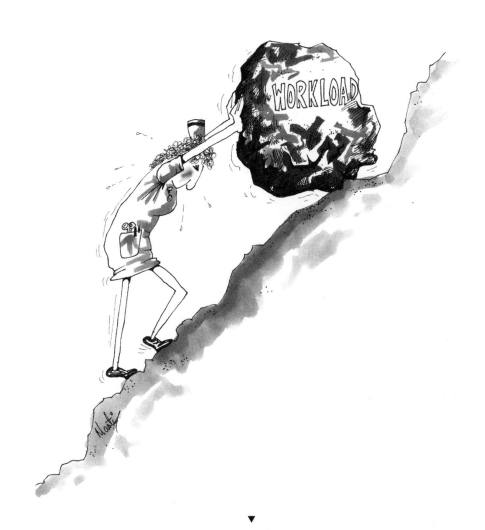

▼

Escalating workload.

Stress and performance at work

There is a common misconception among some managers that efficiency and effectiveness mean achieving more with less. Unfortunately, just like an elastic band that will eventually snap if it has been stretched too far, so an over-stressed workforce will eventually become less effective. In other words, there is an optimum level of demand at which the individual is decisive, creative, working efficiently and effectively. After this point, if a sensible level of demand is exceeded, performance tails off and the individual becomes less effective, less decisive, etc., and eventually becomes exhausted and 'burnt out'.

'Burnout' in health-care workers is known to result in lowered production, increases in absenteeism, increased health care costs and increased personnel turnover.[32] Burnout is recognised as a healthcare professional's occupational disease which must be recognised at an early stage and treated.

Figure 1 below illustrates this sequence of events. The 'fantasy' line shown represents the mental picture that many staff may have of themselves.

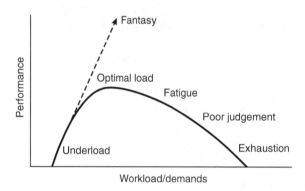

Figure 1: Stress performance curve.

EXERCISE 5   Where are you now? Draw your own stress performance curve.

Now that you have read about the effects of stress on individuals' well-being and performance and studied the standard stress performance curve given here, draw your own stress performance curve below. Will it be a flat curve, or one with a tall peak? Will it be an asymmetrical or symmetrical curve? Fill in at least four positive and four negative adjectives to indicate how the demand/performance ratio affects *you* as a nurse at work.

Draw your own perceived stress performance curve below

Performance

Workload/demands

List four positive adjectives to indicate how your performance is improved by an increased demand on you:

-

-

-

-

List four negative adjectives to indicate how your performance is adversely affected by an increased demand on you:

-

-

-

-

The nurse's response to stress and its effects on individual nurses, colleagues at work and those at home

When a person is confronted with threatening situations, the body has a standard response involving a series of chemical reactions to prepare itself to deal with the emergency by the so-called 'flight or fight' response. However, the way in which people interpret the threat and judge whether or not they can deal with it will vary from one individual to another.

The most common response found among nurses is anxiety. They become anxious about what they are doing, but perhaps more importantly, about what they are unable to do. They worry and become increasingly frustrated. Some, of course, become angry and some may even displace their anger on others, for example by becoming inappropriately angry with patients, junior colleagues, students, or those at home. Alternatively, instead of becoming angry, some individuals withdraw, which eventually leads to apathy and a feeling of helplessness. In addition, others may become easily distracted and feel unable to do anything competently. Indeed, they may feel almost paralysed and trapped, not knowing where to go or what to do next.

When nurses are being prepared for practice, they are constantly reminded of the 'problem-solving' approach to care. With this approach being a core part of their professional repertoire, some nurses may opt for the problem-solving strategy in all situations. In other words, with regard to stress management, they would systematically identify the sources of their stress, realise what effects the stress is having on them, and either find ways to deal with the stress or take action to avoid it. They might argue that staying at home or claiming to be unwell might be one way of avoiding stress, whereas if the source of stress is not dealt with, being absent from work merely postpones the stress until another day. Other nurses might tackle their stress problems either by changing their behaviour, e.g. by engaging in outdoor hobbies or relaxation classes, or by seeking solace in alcohol or drugs.

Although nurse leaders and managers are aware of the potential manifestations of prolonged stress, and are sympathetic to sufferers, they cannot condone behaviour that will contravene the United Kingdom Central Council's (UKCC's) 'Code of Professional Conduct'.[33–35] Some of the poor coping strategies that might be adopted could also get the stressed individual into deeper water and the likelihood of being disciplined or removed from the professional register, such as errors with regard to decision-making or procedures.

The effects of the stress 'virus' on colleagues at work include the following:

1 Poor team spirit

2 Breakdown in communication

3 Too little time for each other, so no deep bonds of friendship or regard are formed

4 Too little support for each other

5 Others feeling stressed by being in the company of the stressed nurse or health professional.

The effects of stress on those at home include the following:

1 Lack of interest in family interests, so that bonds deteriorate

2 One problem creating another (e.g. marital or child's)

3 Lack of support and cohesion

4 Children or spouse feeling that they are unimportant compared to people at work

5 Breakdown of the family unit

6 Preoccupation with work or with people at work.

EXERCISE 6 Where are you now? Compare the effects which you perceive that stress has on you with what other colleagues think about themselves.

To find out what effects of stress at work apply to *you*, fill in the questionnaire in Table 1 below. The effects of stress are not listed in any order of priority. Other health professionals have identified them. Tick whether these are effects of stress for you, ticking 'no', 'somewhat' or 'significant' according to how you perceive that effect. Then rank each effect from 1 to 10 according to how significant an effect it is for you, where '1' is the most significant effect of stress for you and '10' is the least significant. Enter your ranking in the far right-hand column. Then compare your results with those of general practitioners and practice managers from another study,[36] shown in Table 2 below. Please do not worry if your results do not match with theirs, which are simply offered as a baseline for comparison. That is why we have also left blank rows in tables for you to enter the effects of stress that apply *to you in your workplace*.

Table 1

Effect of stress on your workplace	No	Somewhat	Significant	Ranking
Frequent staff turnover				
Thefts				
Mistakes				
Staff turning up late				
Not being able to do much for patients				
Too many staff going off sick				
Poor workplace management				
Arguments or angry outbursts at work				
Poor relationships with patients				
Complaints				

EXERCISE 6   Continued.

Effect of stress on your workplace	No	Somewhat	Significant	Ranking
Poor relationships between staff				
Disloyalty				
Accidents				
Poor decision-making				
Other:				
Other:				
Other:				

Table 2

Effects of stress	GPs' rank order	Practice managers' rank order	Your rank order from questionnaire above
Mistakes	1	1	
Arguments or angry outbursts	2	2	
Poor relationships with patients	3	4	
Poor relationships between staff	4	3	
Increased staff sickness	5	5	
Increased staff turnover	6	6	
Other:			
Other:			
Other:			
Other:			
Other:			

EXERCISE 7   Where are you now? Summarising sources and effects of stress for you.

This exercise will pull together all of the work you have done throughout the Module. By now you should have a good appreciation of the factors related to you, your work, your home situation and your life in general that are causing you stress. In this exercise, look back at your answers given in the first five exercises, and summarise the key causes of stress for you in each of the six categories with respect to how you operate at work and how you function outside work. Write these key causes down in the first column under 'symptoms of stress'. Then decide how these symptoms affect your behaviour, your life, your relationships and your performance at work in the 'outcomes' column. The outcomes will include the end results of these symptoms of stress for you, impinging either directly on you or indirectly from the effects on your organisation. For example, 'mistakes' or 'rows at home' might have the outcome that you lose your job, become estranged from your family or divorce your spouse.

First complete the exercise for how it is *for you at work* in Table A. Then *repeat* the exercise for how it is *for you outside work* in Table B.

Table A

Sources of stress at work	Symptoms of stress (your own and organisational symptoms)	Outcomes for you
To do with the job itself		
Your role in your work setting		
Your relationships at work		
Your career development		
Conflict at your home–work interface		
The organisation or management of your workplace		
The hospital, Trust or general practice organisation itself		

EXERCISE 7   Continued.

Table B

Sources of stress outside work	Symptoms of stress (your own and others' symptoms)	Outcomes for you
To do with your family/home		
Your role at home		
Your relationships with others outside work		
Your career development		
Conflict at your home–work interface		
The community or environment		

And finally

EXERCISE 8   Where are you now? Are you experiencing too much stress? Do you need help?

- Are you experiencing too much stress? Are you determined to act to minimise stress?

- Can you minimise the stresses in your life by yourself, or do you need help?

EXERCISE 8   Continued.

Look back at Exercise 2. If a main cause for you is 'manager's demands' and/or 'too much work', then you should go on to Module 2 (controlling stress) and Module 3 (assertiveness skills).

If a main cause for you is 'patient abuse or aggression' then you should go on to Module 3 (assertiveness skills), which also includes material on combating aggression.

If a main cause for you is 'poor organisation', you need to work through Module 2 (controlling stress) and Module 4 (defining time management).

If a main cause of stress is 'work pressures' you should work through Module 2 (controlling stress), Module 3 (assertiveness skills) and Module 5 (enhancing job satisfaction).

If a main cause of stress for you is 'poor communication', you should go on to Module 2 (controlling stress), Module 5 (enhancing job satisfaction) and Module 6 (promoting career development) to look at other opportunities.

Meantime, what changes can you make:

• Today (name one)?

• Tomorrow (name two, however trivial)?

• Next week (name three, however small)?

References

1 Richards C (1989) *The health of doctors.* King's Fund, London.

2 Clark E, Montague ES (1993) The nature of stress and its implications for nursing practice. In Hinchliff S, Norman S, Schober J (eds) *Nursing practice and health care: a foundation text.* Arnold, London.

3 Headlines (1995) Stress and sickness force nurses to quit. *BMJ.* **311**: 1522.

4 Radford T (1994) White-collar workers turn to chocolate, tea, coffee, alcohol and smoking to cope with worst level of stress in Europe. *The Guardian*, 14 November.

5 Lees S, Ellis N (1990) The design of stress management programmes for nursing personnel. *J Adv Nurs.* **15**: 946–61.

6 Selye H (1976) *The stress of life.* McGraw-Hill, New York.

7 Hingley P, Cooper CL (1986) *Stress and the nurse manager.* John Wiley & Sons, Chichester.

8 Lindop E (1991) Individual stress among nurses in training: why some leave whilst others stay. *Nurse Educ Today.* **11**: 110–20.

9 Parkes K (1985) Stressful episodes reported by first-year student nurses: a descriptive account. *Soc Sci Med.* **20**: 945–53.

10 Arnold J (1989) Experiences and attitudes of learner nurses during their first year of training, Unpublished Report of Manchester School of Management, University of Manchester Institute of Science and Technology, Manchester.

11 Birch J (1979) The anxious learners. *Nurs Mirror.* **148**: 17–22.

12 Baglioni AJ, Cooper CL, Hingley P (1990) Job stress, mental health and job satisfaction among senior nurses. *Stress Med.* **6**: 9–20.

13 Kushnir T (1986) Stress and social facilitation: the effects of the presence of an instructor on student nurses' behaviour. *J Adv Nurs.* **11**: 13–19.

14 Melia KM (1987) *Learning and working: the occupational socialisation of nurses.* Tavistock Publications, London.

15 Cavanagh SJ, Snape J (1993) Nurses under stress. *Senior Nurse.* **13**: 40–2.

16 Field D (1989) *Nursing the dying.* Routledge, London.

17 Vachon ML (1987) *Occupational stress in the care of the critically ill, dying and the bereaved.* Hemisphere, Washington.

18 Doweney V *et al.* (1995) Dying babies and associated stress in NICU nurses. *Neonat Network.* **14**: 41–6.

19 Oates RK, Oates P (1995) Stress and mental health in neonatal intensive care units. *Arch Dis Child.* (fetal and neonatal edition) **72**: 107–10.

20 Thornton S (1984) Caring for special babies. III. Stress in neonatal intensive care units. *Nurs Times.* **80**: 35–7.

21 Rosenthal RH *et al.* (1989) Stress and coping in a NICU. *Res Nurs Health.* **12**: 257–65.

22 Bailey JT, Steffen SM, Grout JW (1980) The stress audit: identifying the stressors of ICU nursing. *J Nurs Educ.* **19**: 15–25.

23 Bibbings J (1987) The stress of working in intensive care: a look at the research. *J Clin Nurs.* **3**: 567–70.

24 Duggan NM (1990) The stress of working in intensive care: a literature review. *Irish Nurs Forum Health Serv.* **8**: 22–3, 25–9.

25 Norrie P (1995) Do intensive care staff suffer more stress than staff in other care environments? A discussion. *Intens Crit Care Nurs.* **11**: 293–7.

26 White D, Tonkin J (1991) Registered nurses' stress in intensive care units: an Australian perspective. *Intens Care Nurs.* **7**: 45–52.

27 Keller KL (1990) Sources of stress and satisfaction in the practice of emergency medicine: a comparative study of nurses and physicians. *J Emerg Nurs.* **16**: 413–14.

28 Hawley MP (1992) Sources of stress for emergency nurses in four urban Canadian emergency departments. *J Emerg Nurs.* **18**: 211–16.

29 Sowney R (1996) Stress debriefing: reality or myth? *Accid Emerg Nurs.* **4**: 38–9.

30 Atkinson LR *et al.* (1996) *Hilgard's introduction to psychology.* Harcourt Brace College Publishers, London.

31 Cox T (1993) *Stress research and stress management: putting theory to work.* Health and Safety Executive, London.

32 Felton JS (1998) Burnout as a clinical entity – its importance in health care workers. *Occup Med.* **48**: 237–50.

33 United Kingdom Central Council for Nursing, Midwifery and Health Visiting (UKCC) (1992) *Code of professional conduct.* UKCC, London.

34 United Kingdom Central Council for Nursing, Midwifery and Health Visiting (UKCC) (1992) *The scope of professional practice.* UKCC, London.

35 United Kingdom Central Council for Nursing, Midwifery and Health Visiting (UKCC) (1996) *Guidelines for professional practice.* UKCC, London.

36 Chambers R, George V, McNeill A, Campbell I (1998) Health at work in the general practice. *Br J Gen Pract.* **48**: 1501–4.

Other reading

Arroba T, James K (1992) *Pressure at work: a survival guide for managers.* McGraw-Hill Book Company, London.

Bailey R (1986) *Coping with stress in caring.* Blackwell Scientific Publications, Oxford.

Bailey R, Clarke M (1989) *Stress and coping in nursing.* Chapman & Hall, London.

Beck J (1984) Nurses have needs too: take time to care for yourselves. *Nurs Times.* **80**: 31–2.

Burnard P (1991) *Coping with stress in the health professions: a practical guide.* Chapman & Hall, London.

Callahan P, Morrisey J (1993). Social support and health: a review. *J Adv Nurs.* **18**: 203–10.

Clarke M (1992) Stress and the individual. In Kenworthy N, Snowley G, Gilling C (eds) *Common foundation studies in nursing.* Churchill Livingstone, London.

Clarke VA, Ruffin CL (1992) Perceived sources of stress among student nurses. *Contemp Nurse.* **1**: 35–40.

Cobbs S (1976) Social support as a moderator of life stress. *Psychosom Med.* **38**: 300–14.

Cochran J, Ganong LH (1989) A comparison of nurses' and patients' perceptions of intensive care unit stressors. *J Adv Nurs.* **14**: 1038–43.

Cohen S, McKay G (1984) Social support, stress and the buffering hypothesis: a theoretical analysis. In Baum A, Taylor S, Singer J (eds) *Handbook of psychology and health.* Erlbaum, New Jersey.

Cox T (1978) *Stress.* Macmillan Press, London.

Fletcher B (1991) *Work, stress, disease and life expectancy.* John Wiley & Sons, Chichester.

Fontana D (1989) *Managing stress.* British Psychological Society and Routledge, London.

Freud A (1946) *The ego and mechanism of defence.* Hogarth Press, London.

Hayward J (1975) *Information: a prescription against pain.* Royal College of Nursing, London.

Hinchliff S, Norman S, Schober J (1993) *Nursing practice and health care: a foundation text.* Edward Arnold, London.

Kenworthy N, Snowley G, Gilling C (1992) *Common foundation studies in nursing.* Churchill Livingstone, London.

Lazarus RS (1966) *Psychological stress and the coping process.* McGraw-Hill, New York.

Lazarus RS (1976) *Patterns of adjustment.* McGraw-Hill, New York.

Lazarus RS, Launier R (1978) Stress-related transactions between person and envoronment. In Pervin M, Lewis M (eds) *Perspectives in interactional psychology.* Plenum Press, New York, pp. 287–327.

Lazarus RS, Folkman S (1984) *Stress, appraisal and coping.* Springer, New York.

Marshall J (1980) Stress among nurses. In Cooper CL, Marshall J (eds) *White-collar and professional stress.* John Wiley & Sons, Chichester.

Patel C (1991) *The complete guide to stress management.* Optima, London.

Power P (1996) High anxiety. *Nurs Times.* **92**: 58.

Rhead MM (1995) Stress among student nurses: is it practical or academic? *J Clin Nurs.* **4**: 369–76.

Snell J (1995). It's tough at the bottom. *Nurs Times.* **91**: 55–8.

Steen L (1994) So you want to be a nurse? *Can Nurse.* **90**: 55.

Sutherland VJ, Cooper CL (1990) *Understanding stress: a psychological perspective for health professionals.* Chapman & Hall, London.

Wilson G (1991) Technology and stress. *Nurs J Clin Pract Educ Manag.* **4**: 31.

Wilson-Barnett J (1979) *Stress in hospital.* Churchill Livingstone, Edinburgh.

Wilson-Barnett J (1986) Reducing stress in hospital. In Tierney A (ed.) *Clinical nursing practice: recent advances in nursing.* Churchill Livingstone, Edinburgh.

Video and relaxation tapes

Videos for Patients Ltd. For videos such as 'Stress': 122 Holland Park Avenue, London W11 4UA. Tel: 0171 229 5161; Fax: 0171 221 3832.

Wendy Lloyd Audio Productions Ltd. For audio-cassette tapes such as the twin tapes of 'Coping with stress at work', 'The relaxation kit' and 'Feeling good': 30 Guffitts Rake, Meols, Wirral L47 7AD. Tel: 0151 632 0662.

MODULE 2
Controlling stress

AIMS

The aims of Module 2 are:

1 To increase nurses' understanding of the range of options and solutions that are likely to control or minimise stress.

2 To actively engage nurses in reducing a major source of stress.

3 To encourage nurses to make a timetabled action plan to reduce the stress in their lives.

4 To help nurses to reduce the effects of their stress on their partner and/or family at home, and their colleagues at work.

CONTENTS

The total time needed to work through the module depends on the amount of time you spend reflecting on how the information in the module applies to you before completing the exercises. The total time it might take to complete this module is 9 hours (including time for reading and thinking and for completing the significant event analyses, stress reduction exercise and timetabled action plans).

Below are the comments that some participants made about what they had gained from previous *Survival Skills* programmes.

'The course has helped to improve my confidence. It has been extremely beneficial to know that others have had similar experiences and anxieties.'

'I felt a very different person when I started this module – I think I was actually quite dangerously stressed, but now I feel more in control.'

'I feel reassured that I'm in the normal range of colleagues.'

'As a result (of doing the first module) I've already made several changes in the last few months to ease my stress.'

'The best part was realising that the feelings I have are those of stress, not a serious illness, and I can work through this.'

'I thought you might like to know what effect the stress management course had. I did take quite a long hard look at both work and personal stress. I decided I was overcommitted and reduced non-essential work drastically, deciding it was pointless having the money but not the energy or time to enjoy it. I reorganised my work times so that they were realistic and I no longer had to "chase myself" because I was running late. There were several other small (but cumulative) changes at work as well. I also joined a leisure club where there are trainers who monitor my progress in the gym (essential for me – to ensure regular attendance) and part of the programme involves relaxation at the end of training. I can take the family there as well. All told, I think the course had a big impact. I do feel much less pressurised. I still get the odd stress-filled day, but changes I have made make it easier to manage.'

'The course helped me look at myself and how I contribute to stresses and how I work towards stopping this.'

'I've started using my diary more to plan my time, and I now feel less pressurised.'

'I enjoyed being made to address my problems and identify ways of reducing my stress levels – for example, I would never have thought of changing my working arrangements without this stimulus.'

'... being made to think what I might do to help myself feel more in control rather than defeated all the time.'

'The programme forced me to look at what I do and the stress it induces, and suggested and reinforced that I can change things.'

'It has taught me things about recognising and coping with stress that I did not know before.'

'Advice is also useful in helping stressed patients.'

'I enjoyed ... (the programme) ... it made me feel hopeful and enthusiastic that I can have some control of the situation.'

REDUCING STRESS EFFECTIVELY: OPTIONS AND SOLUTIONS

There are three types of responses to stress – physiological, psychological and behavioural reactions. The way in which you respond depends on personal factors such as age, gender, personality, previous family and personal experiences, as well as coping ability and other organisational options.

Six characteristics of stressful work are poor status, poor pay, job insecurity and redundancy, low social value, career uncertainty and career stagnation.[1] Most of these are certainly applicable to nursing. On the whole, many nurses do not think out plans to cope with the stresses in their lives and just hope for the best, often preferring avoidance and evasion techniques! Often their struggles to overcome stress and their reluctance to admit they are unable to cope mean that the stress problem becomes even worse.

Surveys of other health professionals have shown that they do not tackle stresses systematically either, and that they put up with the stresses heaped upon them by their colleagues in an unassertive way.[2]

The kind of practical methods that some nurses use to cope with stress at work are as follows:

• seeking support from colleagues/family/friends

• sharing problems with professional colleagues

• adoption of better time management practices

• more appropriate appointment times for patients

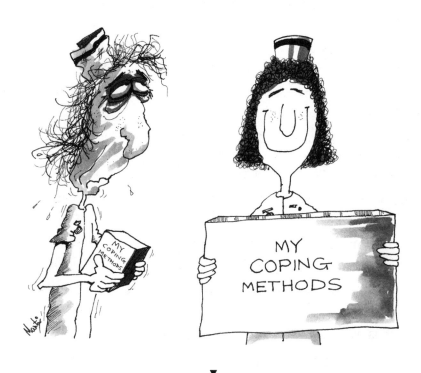

▼

Options and solutions.

- protected off-duty time
- admission of doubts and worries to others
- achieving a better balance between work and home commitments.

It is difficult to make plans to cope with stress more effectively until you understand how you and others around you actually respond to stress. Therefore the next section will explore your own responses to stress at work and home.

Having identified your main causes of stress, you need to make a priority list. Some points on the list will require other colleagues to co-operate with the redistribution of tasks. Changes will have to be negotiated, especially if they involve delegating work or altering other nurses' workloads. Having delegated as many of your stresses as are practicable, you can still expect to retain a hard core which you cannot escape. You will have to devise specific coping strategies in order to overcome or reduce them.

Learn to relax so that you can make the most of any free period, even for only a few minutes. Try and train yourself to shut right off from your surroundings at will. You will need a quiet room where you can be undisturbed, at your workplace or at home, or even in your car.

Avoid the seven deadly sins of the workaholic.

1 Stop being a perfectionist.

2 Don't judge your mistakes too harshly.

3 Resist the desire to control everything.

4 Learn to decline extra commitments assertively if you are already pressed for time.

5 Look after your personal health and fitness.

6 Allow time for personal growth, the family and leisure.

7 Don't be too proud to ask for help.

The pressure for peak performance day after day can lead to burnout, whereas a sensibly planned programme, including protected time, can lead to optimal performance and a more balanced way of life. Let go a little. Too many extra demands are impossible to absorb as opportunities, and you must continually reassess your priorities.

Lower your standards to realistic levels. Stop being a perfectionist and accept being 'good enough'. Have you considered whether you are setting your personal standards too high and aiming for excellence too much of the time? Don't feel guilty about not being the ideal nurse at all times.

Review the degree to which you are in control of your own life at work and home, and how much more control you should try to take. Stop banging your head against a brick wall trying to control things you have no chance of changing. Become more laid back, and reserve your energy for being in control of the things that really matter.

Stress can be either positive or negative, depending on how you perceive it and how you react to it. If you view new regulations as challenges, you will probably find ways of managing such changes to your advantage, with opportunities for learning and growth.

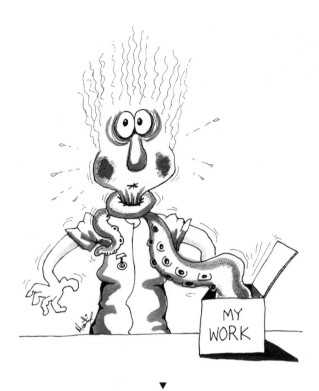

▼

Control over your work?

Look after your health. Some nurses deny their own needs for rest and recuperation, feeling that they are indispensable and playing down their own symptoms of illness. Compare how you behave when you are ill with what most people would do, and try to narrow the gap. Staying fit and healthy involves good physical, mental and spiritual well-being.

Reduce your professional commitments. Be sure of your motives for taking on commitments over and above your core nursing post. If you have just drifted into committee work or felt initially that you could not say 'no', this might be the time for you to weigh up whether those commitments are still worthwhile.

The objective of learning to cope better is to regain a balance between work and the rest of your life. One of the best coping methods of all, therefore, is not to take on the additional task or responsibility in the first place if it is not necessary. Just because you can do something well or find it interesting, or you are flattered to be asked, does not mean that you should take it on when you are already pressed for time or distracted by other pressures.

This may require you to learn assertiveness skills and practise them at every opportunity. Assertiveness is about knowing and practising your rights – to change your mind, to make mistakes, not to understand about something (for example, the complex uses of the computer), to refuse demands, to express emotions, to be yourself without having to act for other people's benefit, and to make decisions or statements without always having to justify them. There is a narrow line between being assertive and behaving in an aggressive, bossy way – sometimes it takes practice to get it right.

Be prepared to ask for help. Seeking support is a coping skill not often employed by nurses, who feel that it may be regarded as a sign of weakness or ignorance. Support networks or clinical supervision may be used to obtain another professional opinion, e.g. between teams or within Trusts, or for emotional assistance. Encouraging nursing colleagues and other members of the team to trust each other over sensitive issues may help to defuse personal worries and stresses enormously. The support from others needs to be non-judgmental and given in an environment where people do not feel embarrassed or silly about asking for help. Specialist and community nurses can feel lonely and isolated at work, and may feel compelled to fit into a culture where they are expected to keep their anxieties and stresses to themselves rather than burden their colleagues.

If a nurse is fortunate enough to have a close and supportive spouse and family at home, that can be a good safe place to offload and share worries about work, so long as doing this does not put too much pressure on personal relationships.

Nurses learn to cope 'no matter what' during pre-registration nurse training, but to carry on uncomplainingly in the face of escalating demands is not right. So talk to your colleagues. Who will understand your worries about patients' complaints or excessive demands better than your work colleagues? If you express your feelings they may state theirs too, and together maybe you can do something about it.

To stay on top, you may need to regain your enthusiasm for learning and your quest for knowledge and understanding. The personal satisfaction that is derived from completing a project, diploma, degree course or some other educational endeavour is likely to make any nurse feel more fulfilled and to reawaken an interest in a wide range of nursing practice. Adopting positive thinking and finding time for personal and professional development are vital.

Nurses are vulnerable to stress because so many of their patients or clients are anxious and stressed about coming into contact with the NHS, and fearful about their complaints. This anxiety, stress and fear can unfortunately be transferred to the nurses and colleagues they are consulting, creating pressure for them unless the nurses and other health professionals are 'stress-proofed' or know how to reduce their own stress levels by developing their own personal strategies.

Don't forget – research into stress has shown that people with the best social supports, who interact well with other people, have the best ability to cope with stress and are the least affected by it. Remember it is not stress itself that is the damaging factor, but your inability to cope with it. In a changing world you need to learn new ways of coping. That way lies survival.

RESPONSES TO STRESS

EXERCISE 1   Where are you now? With whom do you discuss your troubles?

Various types of people with whom a nurse might discuss stress issues, or seek help and advice, are listed below. Put a tick in the column to indicate if you have ever sought advice or discussed ideas for coping with workload, stress or the demands made by work. Add another tick if you have ever considered seeking advice or discussion on these topics with anyone listed. If there are people whom you could have approached but haven't, what has held you back?

	From whom have you ever sought advice or help or discussion?	*From whom would you like to have sought advice, help/discussion?*
Friend(s)		
Colleagues at work		
Spouse/partner or family member		
Own GP		
Clinical supervisor		
Occupational health staff member		
Community psychiatric nurse		
Counsellor		
Mentor		
Manager		
Clergy		
Educationalist, e.g. university lecturer		
Skills course organiser		
Other:		

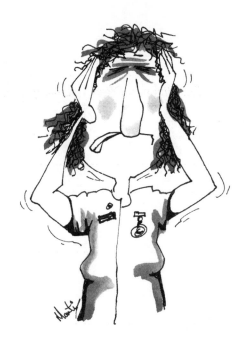
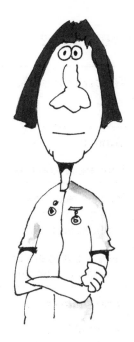

▼

Responses to stress.

One of the membership benefits of belonging to the Royal College of Nursing (RCN) is access to the 'Working Well Initiative' which they publish. If you are facing serious problems at work, your local occupational health department can introduce you to a counsellor who will give you support to help you cope with the emotional traumas. The nursing unions will also help in work-related disputes by offering advice and by conciliating or mediating between both parties.

EXERCISE 2   Where are you now? How do you usually respond to stress?

To reflect on how you usually respond to stress, complete the questionnaire below, which describes different types of responses. The responses listed below are not ranked in any order of priority or of markers of success. They have been identified as ways in which health professionals respond to stress.[2,3] Please score each factor according to how you believe you usually respond (or write N/A if it is not appropriate for you, e.g. if you do not drive a car, so that 'driving at high speed' is not an option). If you usually respond in ways that are not featured in the table, please add them to the bottom of the list. Finally, rank in order of frequency the types of response that you adopt most often.

Response to stress	Never or seldom	Sometimes	Often	Ranking
Seek discussion with colleagues or friends				
Drive at high speed				

EXERCISE 2 Continued.

Response to stress	Never or seldom	Sometimes	Often	Ranking
Overeat				
Feel angry and frustrated				
Passive relaxation (e.g. watching TV, relaxation tape)				
Take a complete break when not on duty				
Seek counselling				
Be irritable with colleagues or patients				
Drink more alcohol				
Take more exercise				
Feel helpless, anxious or depressed				
Manage time better				
Delegate tasks				
Avoid stressful situations				
Have difficulty in concentrating				
Use laughter or jokes				
Drive car fast				
Other:				
Other:				

Other responses might be to reduce caffeine/coffee intake, or to play music, get a pet, take up a new hobby, sleep, pray or practise yoga.

Turn over the page and compare your ranking with that of a group of general practitioners whose coping responses have been studied.[2]

EXERCISE 2 Continued.

General practitioners' ranking of frequency of different responses to stress at work.

Response to stress	GPs' ranking	Your ranking
Take a complete break	1	
Seek discussion with colleagues or friends	2	
Passive relaxation	3	
Use laughter or jokes	4	
Take more exercise	5	
Feel anger towards patients or colleagues	6	
Avoid stressful situations	7	
Drink more alcohol	8	
Manage time better	9	
Overeat	10	
Drive car fast	11	
Be irritable	12	
Delegate tasks	13	
Seek counselling	14	

How similar was the ranking of your usual responses compared with that of these GPs?

There were six 'good' responses in their top ten, but the other four types of response were all of the kind which might make circumstances worse, e.g. drinking more alcohol.

EXERCISE 3   Where are you now? How successful were the work-based coping methods you have tried in the past?

Please tick the column below to indicate which self-help actions you have tried in the past. Was your response or action successful? Note down briefly what happened when you used the coping method (e.g. if you restricted paperwork – how, when and what?). Did the coping method work for you and reduce your stress? Do you still use that coping method?

Coping method	Tried in the past? (Yes/No)	Was it successful? (Yes/Partly/No)
Reduce interruptions		
Decrease workload		
Restrict paperwork		
Plan for extra patients		
Better timed appointments		
Treatment room more comfortable		
Limit the nurse–patient relationship		
Others not mentioned:		

ACTING TO REDUCE STRESS AT WORK

Now that you have read through the synopsis of how nurses cope with stress, and compared your own responses with how other health professionals react to stress, you should have reflected on whether you have been adopting sensible coping methods or just letting pressures mount up as the situation drifted along. Read through the practical steps and tips on a range of coping methods that follow, and then review how you have behaved in the past.

Surveys of stress in nursing uncover a long list of causes – interruptions, workload, paperwork, heartsink patients, patients' or clients' demands, dealing with death and dying, abusive patients, complaints, and so on. In order to minimise stress, you need first to identify the prime causes as in Module 1 of this educational programme, and then to make changes so as to reduce or avoid them.

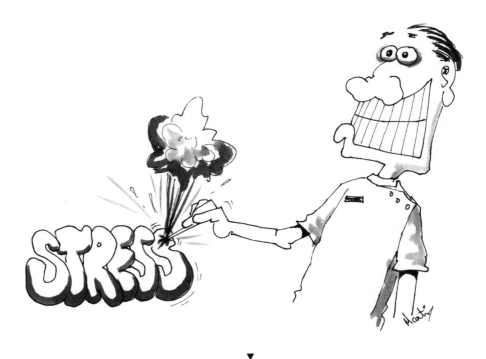

▼

Acting to reduce stress.

Reduce interruptions

People are stressed by situations over which they have little control, such as interruptions. If you go into work early in order to do paperwork, you will get little done and feel increasingly irritated if there are incessant telephone calls or enquiries from colleagues.

- Restrict interruptions at designated times in order to clear your paperwork. Ask colleagues to stall enquiries until you say that you are available.

- Introduce a time when you are available for non-urgent requests.

- Negotiate changing the system to suit you better – but obviously you must be accessible to patients and other staff at some times.

Decrease workload

More work is being undertaken with fewer resources, and patients or clients are becoming more demanding. Your workload is therefore very likely to increase unless you do something about it.

- Consider whether the way in which nursing care is provided or visits are undertaken is appropriate or whether, for example, an appointment system for home visits would be more efficient.

- Decide whether any of the work involved in nursing could be undertaken by others with the appropriate training.

- See what administrative or clerical work could be taken over by other staff. This might mean preparing and submitting a report to your manager highlighting the time spent filing. For example, analysis of one health visitor's working practice identified that there were 114 filing activities associated with providing a normal health-visiting service to one child between birth and five years.

- Reappraise whether you have the right balance between the amount of time you work and your earnings. Consider dropping additional activities or sessions if you are finding your workload too much and you can manage on less money.

Restrict paperwork

- Never handle a letter or report more than once – read it and act on it. If you procrastinate you will waste time rereading it later.

- Complete the most complicated paperwork first when your mind is fresh.

- Carry a tape recorder with you and dictate reminders to yourself to follow up later.

Plan for urgent extra patients

One of the most stressful aspects of working in the community and some acute settings is the number of unexpected extra patients who need to be seen. This is best tackled as a team.

- Everyone will need to agree to a common policy and stick to it.

- There will have to be enough free slots to book same-day appointments for patients or clients who have urgent problems that require to be seen.

- Introducing a protocol which is agreed by all team members may help reduce the number of patients who consider that they need to be seen urgently.

- Whatever changes you decide on, all team members will need to be familiar with the protocol to make it work, so involve them in its development.

Time yourself

Time your work sensibly. If keeping to time is difficult and a major stress for you, consider negotiating with your manager to alter the rate at which you see patients or clients.

If you always end your shift 30 minutes late:

- review the content of your patient contact; are you undertaking nursing activities for 95% of the time, or is some of the time being lost in social chit-chat?

- consider negotiating longer time slots.

Make your workplace as comfortable as possible

This may involve negotiation with colleagues.

- Review your workplace to see how you can make it more comfortable or easier for you to work in.

- Rearrange furniture such as your desk and the chairs, change your chair if it makes your back ache, and obtain another storage cabinet if you want to tidy some of the papers away from view.

- Try a new position for the computer so that it is more accessible, and set up a better system for referral and investigation forms.

- Treat yourself to some little item of luxury that will cheer you up on a bad day – a coffee-maker for use by yourself and your colleagues, a supply of herbal tea bags, a new picture for your wall, or a transistor radio to keep in your office for when you are doing paperwork.

Use visual distraction

- Make sure that there is something visual that is easily seen from your workplace that can be used to distract you when the going gets tough. A photograph of the family is the traditional answer, although photographs of special places or events can work equally well.

- Perhaps a holiday memento that you associate with happy times could be one of the best methods of transporting you from the stresses of nursing and reminding you of the next holiday on your horizon.

Limit the intensity of your relationships with patients

Every nurse knows that the closer the nurse–patient relationship is, the more it drains the nurse. Obviously, if you never interact with your patients and 'give yourself' in any way, your work would be dissatisfying and that could be a source of stress in itself. However, the converse is also true, and you should guard against becoming too involved with your patients' or clients' problems and emotions. Otherwise, you may find that your own family life will suffer as you become emotionally drained, with too little energy and feelings left to give and exchange love and support with your own partner and family.

Nursing can very easily become all-consuming and take priority in nurses' own lives. It is difficult to maintain a distance when working with vulnerable patients whom the nurse knows well and who have serious problems with which the nurse empathises. Somehow, though, nurses have got to learn to maintain a distance and not be sucked into a whirlpool of human emotions and end up devoid of all feeling and burnt out themselves.

Easing the stress on the nurse's family life

No family is immune to the pressures of modern life, and nurses' families may suffer if the nurse parent is worn down by caring for others. The consequences of the pressures on nurses' families will not go away as a result of wishful thinking or ignoring the problems. The pressures need to be examined and somehow faced and, if possible, overcome.

Whatever the causes, if tensions within the family are getting out of hand, the priority is to re-establish better communication. The first step may be to try to distance yourself from your feelings about the situation, and to look from a different viewpoint.

Whole family approach: It sometimes helps to call a family meeting and let everyone have a chance to air their grievances or offer their ideas. Family members need to feel safe enough to speak honestly. But don't have too high expectations at first – they may need time and space to express themselves. This is not a 10-minute assessment, and it is important to abandon the nurse role and become an ordinary family member with good listening skills.

Sharing with your partner: Another approach is to try and inject some freshness into your relationship with your partner. Make a date as in the old days, and try to arrange regular outings for shared activities or interests. Acknowledge any problems with your sex life, if they exist. These are usually due to communication difficulties or lack of time alone together. If you make it a priority and show a little patience, you will probably find some fun and laughter bubbling to the surface.

Enjoying your children: Try to arrange times when your children have your full attention. Talk about your work with them so that they can be more understanding about your being away from home. Try to take more interest in what they are doing, and give more praise when you can. That means overcoming any tendency you might have to praise only academic or sporting success.

Family priorities: It is important to re-evaluate regularly those extra commitments that are keeping you away from the family, especially in the evenings, at night or at weekends, and to see if there are any you might drop or change. Do not regard this as self-sacrifice, but as something you are doing as part of looking after yourself and your family. Get work-related worries off your chest when you come home, and then put them aside. Consider delegating some of the activities which need to be done if you are running a home, working and raising a family. Perhaps employ a cleaner or a gardener, get some help with ironing or decorating, or collaborate with other parents to share the ferrying of children to school and different activities.

Take time out: Plan and take regular holidays. If you and your colleagues have domestic responsibilities which mean that holidays can only be taken at specific times, negotiate at the beginning of each year so that everyone knows what time they are taking and when. The improved quality of life may justify the time spent organising this – ask the family!

Increase the efficiency of your work organisation

If you are to function in as stress-free a way as possible, then you will need to have an efficient and effective work organisation behind you. This could mean reviewing your working practices. You and your colleagues should be well versed in modern theories of management, and communication should be well developed and regarded as being of high priority within the workplace. If you identify problems or potential problems, discuss them with your manager and find out whether you and your colleagues could take advantage of team development opportunities.

Stress reduction can be tackled by a whole team through dedicated courses with subsequent action plans by team members. All staff should know their 'rights' and what is expected of them. Workplace procedures should be made explicit to colleagues and patients or clients in order to minimise any misunderstandings. Complaints policies should be well advertised to colleagues and patients or clients, with the team leader taking the lead with managerial back-up. Work should only be delegated to other staff who have the time and skills to deal with it.

Continuing professional education and participation in clinical supervision are two ways in which to offset the stresses of modern nursing, not only by providing forums for discussion and mutual exchange of worries and solutions, but also by encouraging a life-long philosophy of professional development to cushion nurses against burnout and dissatisfaction with the daily routine.

Relaxation for stress relief

You have to find the method that works best for you. Some people find strenuous exercise more beneficial than deep relaxation. Why not buy or borrow a relaxation tape and see if it is helpful for you? Please do not listen to the tape while driving the car in case it makes you sleepy and less alert than usual. Choose a time and place when you are unlikely to be disturbed, lie back in an armchair or stretch out on a comfortable settee or bed, and play the tape through twice.

This may seem an easy way to manage stress, but it is not. If you are someone who finds it difficult to relax, who becomes fidgety if they are waiting around with nothing to do, you will find that you have to be very firm with yourself in order to listen quietly to the relaxation sessions.

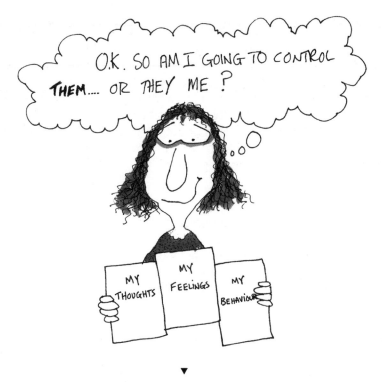

Thoughts + behaviour = stress.

EXERCISE 4   Where do you want to be? What will you do?

Write down below what actions or forms of self-help you intend to use in the near future to control stress. When will you start it?

Proposed self-help action	Start date
1	
2	
3	
4	
5	
6	

Undertaking Significant Event Analyses of Stressful Events

Next time you have an unusually stressful day at work or there is a critical incident in which stress was the trigger factor or result, sit down, reflect and analyse what were the causes and consequences of the stress. When you have done this in relation to an incident connected with your work, repeat the exercise for an extremely stressful event which occurred outside work.

To demonstate this, here are two worked examples.

Analyse a significant event at work

STAGE 1: Write down a factual account of the stressful situation you have chosen – who was involved, at what time of day, and what task/activity you or others were engaged in.

For example, Sister Jones, a practice nurse, became extremely annoyed after a morning session when 10 unexpected extra patients had been added to her appointment list, and she had angrily asked the receptionists why this had occurred. This had made her late for her lunch break, during which she had arranged a dental appointment. So those involved would be Sister Jones, the receptionists, and the patients who overheard the heated discussion.

STAGE 2: Deduce the reasons for the crisis or stressful situation arising for your own case.

In this example, these were disorganised booking of appointments with insufficient capacity for 'extras', and poor communication. Sister Jones had not informed the practice manager of her prior commitment.

STAGE 3: Record the effects of stress on the participants in the crisis or stressful situation you have chosen.

In this example, Sister Jones was even later, left for her dental appointment feeling angry and had difficulty co-operating once there. The practice manager and other staff took sides with the receptionist with whom Sister Jones had been annoyed, and were very aggrieved that Sister Jones had been so unfair. The receptionist at whom Sister Jones had shouted felt humiliated in front of the watching, waiting patients.

STAGE 4: Write down how you or others might have behaved differently, or how the procedures in respect of your designated work might be changed so as to reduce or eliminate the cause of stress.

In this instance, Sister Jones could have told the practice manager about her need to attend the dentist. The practice booking arrangements should be changed to allow sufficient spare capacity for extras. Sister Jones should agree to discuss any organisational problems or concerns with the practice manager in a private room.

Now analyse a significant event outside work

STAGE 1: Write down a factual account of the stressful situation you have chosen – who was involved, at what time of day, and the task/activity you or others were engaged in.

For example, Charge Nurse Edwards came home far later than he had promised to find that his partner was in tears and his children had already left with a friend's parent for the school play in which they were acting.

STAGE 2: Write down the reasons for the crisis or stressful situation arising from your specific situation.

In this example, Charge Nurse Edwards was late because the shift had ended later than planned, the last hour being really hectic, with three new admissions. He was then made later still when the ward clerk asked him to sort out problems with several repeat prescriptions. Then he had had to reorganise the off-duty for the next day because another nurse had broken her arm. But, to be honest, he had forgotten about the school play and the fact that he had promised to go and see it.

STAGE 3: Write down the effects of stress on the participants in the crisis or stressful situation you have chosen.

In this instance, Charge Nurse Edwards' children thought he cared more about his work than them (and they were right!), and because it had happened to them so many times before they were cold-hearted about the situation, and the bond with their father was weakened even further. Charge Nurse Edwards' wife was upset, being torn between loyalty to her husband, acknowledging the importance of his job, and the needs of her children; this was another stage in her increasing feelings of resentment towards her husband for putting his family last. Charge Nurse Edwards was secretly glad he'd got out of going to the school play, but was dismayed to find he had to comfort his wife and show yet another human being some sympathy and kindness, just when he thought he'd left his patients behind and could turn that sort of behaviour off for the day.

STAGE 4: Record how you or others might have behaved differently, or how the work–home interface might be changed so as to reduce or eliminate the cause of stress you have nominated.

In this instance, Charge Nurse Edwards could have prioritised his family's needs and arranged to return home in plenty of time, leaving spare minutes for any unforeseen eventuality at work. He could have changed his shift, told the ward clerk he would sort out the repeat prescriptions in the morning, and delegated the off-duty problem to the next shift leader. The family need not make changes as they could rightfully expect Charge Nurse Edwards' attendance at the school play.

EXERCISE 5   Now undertake your own significant event audit of stress at your workplace, and another for a stressful event arising outside work.

Analyse a significant event at work

STAGE 1: Write down a factual account of the stressful situation you have chosen – who was involved, the time of day, and the task or activity you or others were engaged in.

STAGE 2: Write down the reasons for the crisis or stressful conditions arising from your specific situation.

STAGE 3: Write down the effects of stress on the participants in the crisis or stressful situation you have chosen.

STAGE 4: Record how you or others might have behaved differently, or how the procedures at work might be changed to reduce or eliminate this cause of stress.

EXERCISE 5   Continued.

Then plan for a significant event outside work

STAGE 1: Write down a factual account of the stressful situation you have chosen – who was involved, the time of day, and the task or activity you or others were engaged in.

STAGE 2: Write down the reasons for the crisis or stressful conditions arising from your specific situation.

STAGE 3: Write down the effects of stress on the participants in the crisis or stressful situation you have chosen.

STAGE 4: Record how you or others might have behaved differently, or how the practice/home organisation might be changed to reduce or eliminate your designated cause of stress.

FINDING YOUR OWN SOLUTIONS

Only you can identify the best solutions for you! It may help to decide which stress-reducing interventions you want to make, to classify interventions as being in the following categories:

- *preventive* – that is, you will reduce or change the nature of the stressor, remove the 'hazard' or reduce the frequency or extent of the stressor

- *secondary* – that is, you will alter your own individual response to stress or improve your own or your organisation's ability to recognise and deal with stress-related problems as they arise

- *tertiary* – that is, you will minimise the effects of stress, or help colleagues to cope with and recover from problems arising from stress at work.

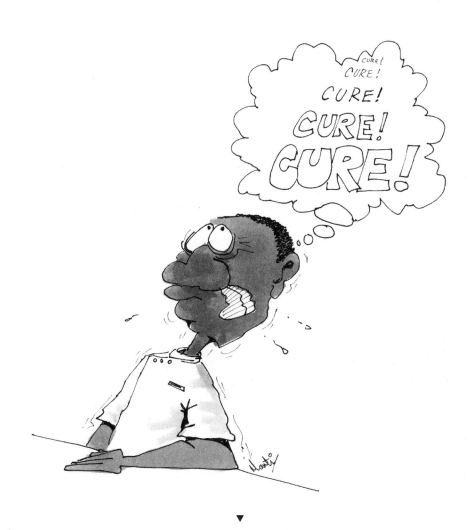

▼

Finding your own solutions.

EXERCISE 6   Where do you want to be and how are you going to get there? Finding your own solutions.

Will you reduce stress at:

• an organisational level in your workplace?

• a team level to support your colleagues?

• your own individual level to improve the way in which you manage work and react to stress?

STAGE 1: Choose which cause of stress you wish to tackle first as an individual, a work team or as an organisation.

This should be a frequent source of stress, an important cause of stress, an infrequent stress which – when it occurs – has far-reaching effects, or a stress which is costly in terms of time or resources. It must be a realistic choice, i.e. a cause of stress which you can reasonably expect to be able to reduce.

The cause of stress for .... is ....

STAGE 2: Set a 'standard' agreed with others from your team/organisation/published literature, or pick a sensible target to aim at (i.e. a goal that is a recognisable measurement of an acceptable lower level of the stress you hope to achieve after you have introduced a new system to reduce the cause of that stress).

You may need to carry out baseline data collection first in order to provide sufficient information to set the standard if there is no obvious reference point. Standards might be agreed levels of personal well-being, time measurements, amount of work delegated, new system(s), work procedures, extent of communication in the team, etc.

The standard is ....

STAGE 3: Write out a plan to reduce the stress, including the expected outcomes and the expected benefits and disadvantages. Discuss your proposal with everyone else involved, at home and at work. Obtain the agreement of anyone who may be concerned about the proposed changes to your set standard(s) and your proposed intervention(s). Amend your plans in the light of others' comments. This stage may include negotiating for and obtaining or buying any extra equipment, training yourself or others if new skills are required, applying for extra staff time, or making other resource or organisational arrangements.

EXERCISE 6   Continued.

Planned intervention is:

Resources needed are:

Expected benefits are:

Expected drawbacks are:

Expected outcomes are:

STAGE 4: Record current performance as a baseline before making any changes.

STAGE 5: Introduce and carry out the intervention. Record the new performance measures.

STAGE 6: Compare the new performance with the old performance, and with pre-set standards. Has the agreed standard been reached?

Feed back information about comparison of performance, outcomes of intervention(s) and the improvements or changes achieved to those involved in or affected by the project. Agree and make further changes if standards were still not met. Negotiate and arrange further training, etc., if your current skills are still inadequate.

STAGE 7: Monitor your performance, including your well-being, 3 to 6 months later. Reinforce interventions and/or changes, etc., as necessary.

And finally

Armed with the knowledge of what seems to cause you the most stress at work and at home (from your daily stress logs computed in Module 1), and what the effects of those stressors are (from your completed questionnaires and your own stress performance curve in Module 1, and the significant event audits in this Module), you are now in a position to make plans to reduce the stresses in your life.

EXERCISE 7   Specify exactly what you intend to do, why, when and how. Choose three more key sources of stress for you, and make plans to tackle them in the near future.

1

2

3

For each source, use the following framework and make a timetabled action plan.

1 What stress will you tackle?

2 Why have you chosen this particular source of stress?

3 What will you do?

4 When will you do it?

5 What other changes will you need to make or what resources will you need to buy?

6 Will the changes involve altering how other people do things?

7 What are the likely benefits to you or your organisation?

8 Are there any drawbacks?

9 What do you expect to be the outcome(s) of your plan?

References

1 Cox T (1993) *Stress research and stress management: putting theory to work.* Health and Safety Executive Contract Research Report No. 61, University of Nottingham, Nottingham.

2 Chambers R, Wall D, Campbell I (1996) Stresses, coping mechanisms and job satisfaction in general practitioner registrars. *Br J Gen Pract.* **46**: 343–8.

3 Wheeler H (1997) Nurse occupational stress research. 3. A model of stress for research. *Br J Nurs.* **6**: 944–9.

Other reading

Arroba T, James K (1992) *Pressure at work. A survival guide for managers.* McGraw-Hill Book Company, London.

Burnard P (1991) *Coping with stress in the health professions.* Chapman & Hall, London.

Cavanagh S, Snape J (1993) Nurses under stress. *Senior Nurse.* **13**: 40–2.

Clark E, Montague ES (1993) The nature of stress and its implications for nursing practice. In Hinchcliff S, Norman S, Schober J (eds) *Nursing practice and health care: a foundation text*, 2nd edn. Edward Arnold, London.

Kennedy P (1997) High pressure areas. *Nurs Times.* **93**: 24–8.

Patel C (1991) *The complete guide to stress management.* Optima, London.

Wheeler H (1997) Nurse occupational stress research. 2. Definition and conceptualization. *Br J Nurs.* **6**: 710–13.

Woodham A (1995) *Beating stress at work.* Health Education Authority, London.

Video and audio-cassette tapes

Videos for Patients Ltd. For videos such as 'Stress': 122 Holland Park Avenue, London W11 4UA. Tel: 0171 229 5161; Fax: 0171 221 3832.

Wendy Lloyd Audio Productions Ltd. For audio-cassette tapes such as the twin tapes of 'Coping with stress at work', 'The relaxation kit' and 'Feeling good': 30 Guffitts Rake, Meols, Wirral L47 7AD. Tel: 0151 632 0662.

MODULE 3
Asserting yourself

AIMS

The aims of Module 3 are:

1 To remind nurses of the advantages of assertive behaviour.

2 To encourage nurses to adopt assertive behaviour.

3 To engage readers in developing and practising assertiveness skills.

CONTENTS

The total time needed to work through this module will depend on the amount of time you spend reflecting on how the information in the module applies to you, before completing the exercises. The total time that it might take to complete this module is 6 hours, including time for reading, thinking and completing all of the exercises.

Below are the benefits that some participants said they had gained from undertaking previous *Survival Skills* programmes:

'I found the section on assertiveness and self-esteem particularly helpful.'

'I had to read and do all of it – hence look at some issues I find unpalatable.'

'It has given me insight and foundations at looking into and identifying my own strengths.'

'The module has been much *better* than expected, and made me realise that the feelings I have are felt by others too, but we don't admit it to each other.'

'What I liked is the idea that you can have a handle on events and emotions.'

'I hadn't realised the differences between being assertive and being aggressive before doing this programme.'

'I used to think that being assertive meant getting other people to agree to doing what you wanted.'

WHAT IS BEING ASSERTIVE ABOUT?

Being assertive is about expressing your feelings clearly and openly and behaving in keeping with those feelings in an honest way. Being assertive is not the same as being aggressive. It is about deciding what you want to do or to happen, judging whether it is reasonable or not, and acting accordingly.

A nurse's natural instinct is to help people, and even those who are hopelessly overworked will often take on extra tasks when they know it is crazy to do so. Assertiveness in the work context is about facing up to the fact that everybody has a limit to their time and energy, and politely but firmly refusing to take on extra work if you know that it will cause you to be over stretched. It is about refusing to be manipulated by others.

Assertiveness is certainly not about getting what you want all the time, nor is it about being a perfectionist and driving yourself and others into the ground. It is about setting out your own boundaries, and being prepared to stick up for yourself if you think you are right while at the same time being willing to reach a compromise with others. You should be able to learn skills to negotiate assertively with everybody – patients, senior and junior colleagues, and family members. It is about giving and taking in an equitable way.

You are not perfect at everything you do. You can use assertiveness to acknowledge your areas of weakness, and then plan to move forward with a particular activity or development.

To be successful at being assertive you have got to understand the tricks that others employ to get their own way. Some patients can be devious, dropping hints about what they really want but placing the onus on you to decide exactly what it is. This is ridiculous. You have better things to do with your time and energy than play these kinds of games. Faced with this type of patient, state clearly and simply what you think is the best way forward, and refuse to be side-tracked. If the patient tries to blackmail you, for example, by saying 'well, you know best, but I do hope I don't have to bother you again later', stick to your guns.

If people try to bully you, and persist even after you have told them 'no', do not give in. Giving in just for some peace and quiet will make things a hundred times worse, and you will feel resentful as well as stressed. Keep saying, calmly but firmly, 'I don't think you heard me, I'm not prepared to do that.' It is important to resist the temptation to get angry. Disarm the anger of a patient or colleague by acknowledging their feelings and staying calm, but do not give in.

Passive behaviour in others can be especially difficult to handle, as it is a technique that nurses may fall for, not liking to appear to take advantage of someone when he or she is down. You are made to feel selfish if you ignore the 'victim's' wishes or hesitant requests. Be careful. You might end up doing what the passive person wants you to do, rather than live with the guilt of pleasing yourself. Respond by stating specifically what you want with a simple explanation. When the next patient needles you, saying 'no one really cares any more about how people feel' or 'I expect it's all my fault', and you feel yourself tempted to reassure them to the contrary, think of the game that they are playing. They are trying to manipulate you. Don't fall for it!

One of the characteristics of someone who is healthily assertive is that they are not afraid to express their opinion. No one should be afraid to give their opinion on a subject they know something about.

Not only do you have as much right to be heard as anybody else, but you also have the right to change your mind. If you decide that, on reflection, you do not want to take on a task, don't be afraid to say so.

The potential advantages for you of being assertive are:

- increased self-confidence

- increased control over your emotions

- the establishment of better relationships with others – people relate to assertive people more readily than to those who are passive or aggressive

- increased self-respect

- increased respect from others

- being more likely to achieve satisfactory changes in your work or home situations.

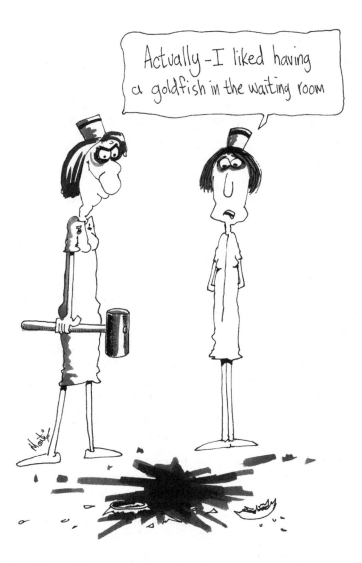

PASSIVE BEHAVIOUR

DOESN'T PAY OFF!

▼

Being assertive.

How assertive are you now?

How do you generally behave at work?

- Passively, just letting things happen to you without letting your feelings be known.

- Assertively, stating clearly what you want and/or how you feel.

- Being abrasive, aggressive or overbearing in order to arrange things the way you want them to be, without regard or respect for other people's feelings and views.

EXERCISE 1   Reflect on how you would usually behave and feel in the following situations:

1 Your manager instructed you to cancel your holiday as another nurse had just gone off sick with stress. Do you think you would:

  a Keep your head down, work harder than ever and say nothing, but seethe inside?

  b Arrange an urgent meeting with the manager to plan other options of how the absent nurse's work might be covered, rather than you having to cancel your holiday?

  c Bawl out anyone giving you extra work, and vent your feelings about the nurse being off sick when everyone else is just as stressed?

2 You are really looking forward to an evening out tomorrow to hear a concert. You will finish work at about 5.00 pm with plenty of time for a leisurely bath before leaving with your partner to hear the performance. Suddenly your plans are dashed. A slip of paper is hurriedly thrust into your hand telling you that you have to change shift tomorrow and work late as your nurse colleague has an important meeting at the Health Authority. Do you:

  a Go home apologetically and say that you will be late tomorrow and will have to cancel your outing to the concert?

  b Explain to the perpetrator of the note that you recognise that the reason for the meeting is important, that you are usually willing to help out, but are unable to do so tomorrow?

  c Storm up to your nurse colleague and disrupt her work by broadcasting your views on the matter and yelling at her?

3 You are quietly getting on with paperwork while there is a lull in your clinical work. Ellen the cleaner comes to your desk and looks as if she wants to chat. She is terribly apologetic, she knows she is a trouble to you and she shouldn't be bothering you with her problems when you are so busy, but she has been having a lot of headaches and all sorts of other aches and pains and wants to know if you think they sound serious. Do you:

  a Stop doing your paperwork and sit and listen to her chattering away, as that is the easiest option?

  b Explain that you have to finish your paperwork, but can meet her for a coffee in the staff rest-room later?

  c Gesture angrily to her to go away, and tell her that you are far too busy to be bothered with her now?

Code: a = passive or unassertive; b = assertive; c = aggressive.

Was your response to these scenarios generally 'passive or unassertive', 'assertive' or 'aggressive'? These might seem to be extreme examples of each type of behaviour, but I expect you can recognise traits in yourself as being likely to mean that you usually behave passively, assertively or aggressively under these kinds of conditions.

Non-verbal behaviour: the body language that gives you away

Passive	Assertive	Aggressive
Covers mouth with hand	Direct eye contact	Gesticulates expansively
Looks down at the floor	Head erect	Clenched/pounding fists
Constant shifting of weight	Descriptive hand gestures	Finger pointing
Fiddles with clothing or jewellery	Emphasises key words	Hands on hips
Rubs head or parts of body	Steady, firm voice	Rigid posture
Frequent nodding of head	Open movements	Strident voice
Throat clearing	Relaxed	Stares others down

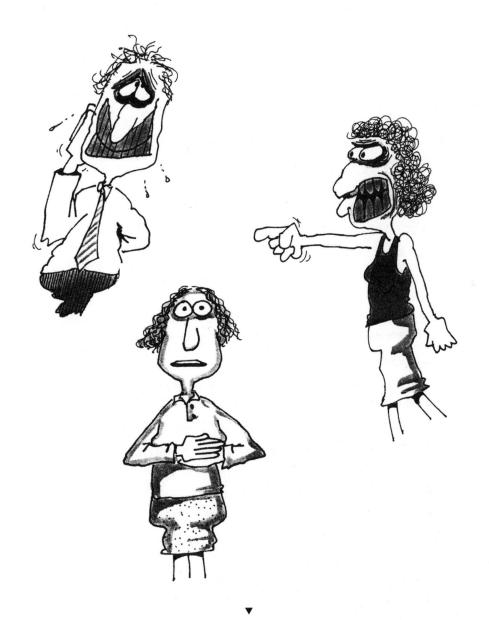

▼

Passive/aggressive/assertive.

What you can do to be more consistently assertive

1 **To be treated with respect**

- Tell others what you want and need, what you like and don't like, and express positives first and negatives second.

- Take pride in your appearance and believe in yourself.

2 **To have and express feelings and opinions**

- Use the 'broken-record' technique, calmly repeating your original statement (at an appropriate time and place).

- Let others know what you are feeling; your vulnerability and trust in others will encourage them to confide in you, too.

3 **To be listened to and taken seriously**

- Match your body language to your assertive message, i.e. stay calm and serious, avoid frivolous quips and use direct eye contact.

- Back up your proposals with well thought out reasons for changes.

- Initiate and get involved in conversations, don't wait for others to approach you first.

4 **To set your own reasonable priorities**

- Set your own goals; dismantle barriers to achieving your goals.

5 **To say 'no' without feeling guilty**

- Use simple, direct language.

- Deflect other people's attempts at distracting you from your purpose; acknowledge that you have heard the other person's viewpoint and repeat your response.

- Distance yourself from problem situations until you get a handle on what's going on, and can be adequately prepared with a considered response.

- Do not lose your self-control and become angry or ill-tempered.

6 **Choose not to assert yourself**

- Try 'active listening': listen, clarify, summarise and paraphrase a speaker's words in order to improve your understanding of their meaning and your rapport.

7 **View your needs as being as important as those of others**

- Learn to recognise the control tactics others are using and be ready to counter them; interrupt back, use flattery, engage them as advisers, or ask for information if you are excluded from a conversation by cryptic remarks.

Tips for assertiveness

1 Say 'No' clearly and then move away or change the subject. Keep repeating 'No', and don't be diverted.

2 Be honest and direct with everyone.

3 Don't apologise or justify yourself more than is reasonable.

4 Offer a workable compromise and negotiate an agreement that suits you and the other party.

5 Pause before answering a 'Yes' you will regret. Delay your response and give yourself more time to think by asking for more information.

6 Be aware of your body language and keep it as assertive as possible. Match your tone to your words (don't smile if you are giving a serious message).

7 Use the 'broken-record' technique, persistently repeating your message in a calm manner to someone who is trying to pressurise you to do something you don't want to do. Don't be side-tracked.

8 Show that you are listening to the other person's point of view and giving them a fair hearing.

9 Practise expressing your opinion and rights rather than expecting other people to guess what you want.

10 Don't be too hard on yourself if you make a mistake – everyone is human.

11 Be confident enough to change your mind if that is appropriate.

12 It can be assertive to say nothing.

Keep practising assertiveness until it comes naturally. Other people are often unaware of their own behaviour, and making an assertive response to an aggressive person may make them realise how they have been behaving. Be aware that if you are angry, it is unlikely that you will manage to be assertive. Challenge people who are sulking, and invite them to tell you if they have a problem. If they deny that they have a problem, treat them normally and don't mention the matter again.

EXERCISE 3   Working through the stages of assertiveness.

Think of an example of a situation at work that occurred in the last few days in which you behaved passively or aggressively, and wish you had been more assertive.

Describe the situation:

Who was involved?

Where did the event happen?

What triggered the episode?

How did you behave? Were you pushy, shy, obnoxious or uncompromising?

How did the other person respond?

How well did you communicate your feelings?

Did you handle any conflict well?

What was the outcome of the exchange?

What should you have done or said?

EXERCISE 4   What are your views on the appropriateness of being assertive with others at work and outside work?

Do you think that there are any disadvantages to being assertive?

Do you have any reservations about becoming more assertive?

List below the people at work or outside work with whom you now intend to be more assertive, and what you expect the outcome(s) to be:

Intend to be more assertive with	Likely outcome(s)
1	
2	
3	
4	
5	

PROMOTING YOUR MESSAGE OR NEGOTIATING YOUR CAUSE ASSERTIVELY

This section gives some practical advice on using assertive behaviour to:

- promote a new message or cause

- negotiate new working conditions or gain other people's co-operation in starting up a new activity.

Promote your message or cause assertively

If you want to change the way in which a section of your organisation works, introduce a new initiative, or persuade others to support your ideas, you will be most likely to succeed in promoting your message or cause by planning out every stage of your 'mini-campaign' and using an assertive approach. There will be plenty of opportunities in the near future, as nurses have higher profiles in primary care groups and Trusts, for getting your message across about a particular cause or way of working that is dear to your heart.

If you hector or bully work colleagues into doing what you want, you might get superficial agreement to your plans and ideas, but you will not achieve their lasting commitment and successful change in the long term. Aggression does not pay off in the end.

You might mistakenly think that, as a nurse, you can have little say in influencing the organisation for which you work. However, you will be surprised what changes you can achieve if you have enough passion about a topic and the persistence to carry your ideas through. This section should provoke your thoughts on the lateral thinking required to put a new message across or start up a new activity that affects and involves others. You will develop your own individual perspective on how best you can influence change: everyone has their own style. Value yours.

Know yourself well

- Understand your own motivation for instigating the change and whether it is really altruism or self-promotion of your ideas (be ready for critics).

- Know your strengths and weaknesses, and your preferred style. Do you understand your own personality profile? Are you an extrovert or an introvert? Whichever it is, select settings in which you are comfortable and perform well – such as committee meetings, networking with others, speaking on the local radio, one-to-one exchanges, or presenting at local professionals' meetings.

- Decide if the message is important enough to be worth the effort. Your passion for the cause will have to motivate you for months or years to come. Your genuineness will show and help to sell your message.

- Be aware of your effect on people. Then you can either deflect their criticisms or rationalise their support or hostility.

- Get into the way of thinking that you can do anything if you want to do so enough – you don't need money to start; you are your own resource.

- Don't be a perfectionist – there's not time.

- Protect yourself from emotional overload. You will get 'sad' cases who try to latch on to your strength – set your own boundaries and be assertive. Don't feel guilty that you cannot help everybody. If you choose a central organisational role to promote your message, you cannot offer many individuals succour as well.

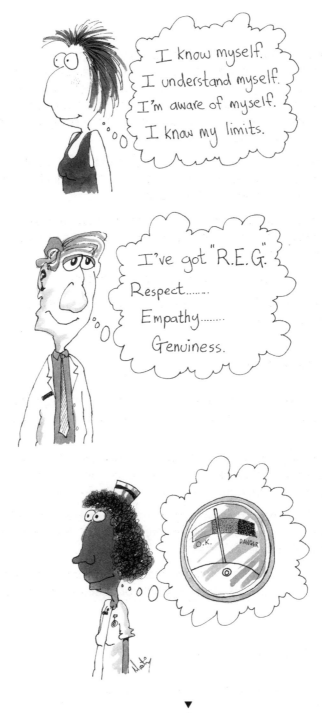

▼

Know yourself.

- Remember that everyone doesn't have to like you.

- Don't let adulation and meeting the 'nobs' (if either apply!) go to your head – you are still just you and a small cog in a mammoth wheel.

- Don't expect admiration, thanks or acknowledgement. There is a lot of jealousy, hostility and backbiting out there if you appear to be successful. Your self-worth and achievement of the tasks you set yourself will have to keep you going. A few faithful colleagues or family members are all that is needed, but they are vital.

Prepare well

- Prepare well for any meeting. Try to make sure that the item you are interested in is towards the top of the agenda (unless you want it to be nodded through when everyone is tired!). Circulate briefing papers before the meeting, and have the answers ready to any queries that might arise, so that the meeting can agree an action plan and not postpone decision-making until more information is available.

- Don't be caught out, whether it is a radio broadcast, local meeting, or an enquiry in the corridor or street. Get training in skills you lack – writing, speaking, using audiovisual aids, broadcasting.

- Do your homework thoroughly first, to develop your key message, so that it rests on a sound and valid base and you won't be taken unawares if new facts come to light.

- Find out the names of people at the top if writing letters.

- Keep good notes about the people you contact, their activities, aspirations and plans for the future.

Deliver your message clearly

- Be consistent – keep giving out the same message, with repetitive sound bites, as the politicians do. Decide early on key words and messages; be faithful to your own style.

- Deliver your message as appropriate for your colleagues, audience or readership – the right words (level and 'language'), in tune with their culture, showing how your cause or change will benefit them.

- Avoid jargon – if you have been mixing with a new group of people you may unconsciously adopt some of their sayings which may grate on your colleagues back at your workplace.

- Whenever possible, leave something about you or your message behind when you talk or meet people, e.g. handouts or business cards – have some with you.

Deliver your message consistently

- Be persistent … follow people up … send them reminders of your work … again … and again …

- Don't waste effort. If you prepare a handout, use it for an article. Practise good time management, and do tricky writing when your mind is fresh and keen.

- Don't duplicate others' work, but build on it. Collaborate so long as you don't end up doing the work for others.

Deliver your message cleverly

- Tackle the promotion of your cause or message from different angles, or through different disciplines.

- Stay in touch and continue to find new material. Update your basic message and ways of promoting it or tangential issues (but not detracting from the basic message). Be creative and surprise people.

- Find ways to orchestrate a 'campaign' or momentum that uses others to promote your message. You will not have much influence as one solitary voice.

- Find out who has the power or is important, and work out ways to influence them. How do they think? What do they need? Can you supply it? Can you give them what they need without making enemies?

- Don't criticise people thoughtlessly – you might be wrong so find out more. Your criticisms might alienate people who could help you to promote your message. On the other hand, don't take any unjustified remarks about you or your interests lying down.

- Gather enough resources by hook or crook to have an assistant to support you, take messages, gatekeep, etc.

Accept credit where credit is due

- Never deny that you are an 'expert' (who is?). Always accept other people's praise – it is only superficial anyway, and they may be saying the opposite tomorrow. Don't be humble – they are lucky that you exhaust yourself promoting the cause, and there is probably no one else apart from you who knows more about it (even if that's too little in your own estimation).

- Don't let others take credit for what you have done – put your name on everything. Send original copies to anyone senior who you think might not realise where the work has come from. Attend all important functions to which you are invited, as far as your diary will let you.

- Don't get too tired of your message; have other interests, too. They will be likely to be 'up' when other issues or feedback are 'down'. Variety keeps you zingy.

- How you promote your message depends on what it is, your circumstances and your own style. You have to find your own way, reflecting on your progress as you go.

EXERCISE 5   Plan out how you might promote a new cause that others around you do not instantly embrace.

You want to set up a self-help support group among your colleagues. No one has ever mooted such a move at your workplace before. You don't know for sure, but you think the idea will be scorned when you first introduce it. How should you go about the challenge of establishing such a group? Map out brief answers to the following framework:

1 What is your motivation for setting up such a group for colleagues?

2 Why should it be you who is involved or organises it?

3 How will you prepare for the challenge of setting up a peer support group?

4 What will your key message be?

5 How and where will you deliver your message?

6 How will you influence other colleagues at work?

7 What is your action plan?

Examples of answers to the challenge of how to go about setting up a peer support group:

• What is your motivation?

EXERCISE 5 Continued.

You believe in the benefits that a peer support group will bring to encourage nurses to devise and follow professional development plans.

- Why should it be you that is involved or organises the group?

No one else has the vision or commitment to organise such an initiative.

- How will you prepare for the challenge of setting up a peer support group?

Find out what others have done in nursing or with different health disciplines. Phone up the managers of any such groups elsewhere and find out what works well and what does not. Look in the local medical or nursing library for help – any literature, experienced facilitator, resources.

- What is your message?

Think out the potential benefits to everyone in the workplace or district – the nurses themselves, their employers and the patients. Prepare your case accordingly, giving an honest appraisal of the advantages and drawbacks.

- How will you deliver your message?

Plan the preliminary information needed to seed your ideas around your workplace and other nursing settings. Follow the usual procedures for introducing new ideas – put it on the agenda for the next staff meeting, write a short article inviting interest in a local newsletter.

- What is your action plan?

A timetabled programme should include details of how to involve all concerned, when and where the meetings will be held, who will be coming, and how costs will be met.

Develop assertive negotiating skills

Negotiating is an integral part of assertive behaviour that is used to reach an agreement that is mutually acceptable to both sides. For instance, you might need to negotiate with a manager or senior colleagues to improve your terms and conditions, or alternatively with junior colleagues or other staff about one of their concerns.

Prepare your arguments well, using logic based on facts and figures rather than offering veiled threats or empty promises. Give a fair assessment of the current situation, not exaggerating or minimising the problems, issues or challenges involved.

You will need to be clear about your objectives in any negotiations, however minor. If you are negotiating for others, you will need a clear brief from them to be sure that their objectives coincide with yours, and how far you are mandated to go on their behalf. You must not exceed their brief, or you may find that you have negotiated an unworkable new arrangement that others disclaim.

State your most important requirements clearly in a straightforward manner. Describe the benefits for the other party – if it is a new scheme at work it might be more clinically effective, more cost-effective or more convenient for doctors, staff or patients.

Listen carefully to the other person's viewpoint, and seek to understand their position and concerns. Clarify what they are saying, their position and the exact terms and conditions that they are offering. Summarise what you think they have just said in order to check out the wording and ensure that there are no ambiguities. Ask open questions to obtain information, and find out what their 'bottom line' is. Look for weaknesses or unfairness in their arguments.

Avoid confrontation or a stalemate by offering other options which you have worked out beforehand as being acceptable alternative solutions. Discuss how each party might trade concessions to reach an acceptable agreement; if the other person makes a concession, don't crow. It is important for the negotiations to remain amicable to avoid loss of face to either party. Give the other person time to reflect on your request, and work through your suggested ideas or changes, rather than demanding an instant response.

Once an agreement is reached, close the discussion. Ruminating back through the problems or different options will only be time-wasting, and the other party may try and reopen negotiations or backtrack on your agreement.

EXERCISE 6   Practise negotiating over an issue you care about now.

Think of something that you have been wanting to change at work and that you have not yet discussed with the others. You should expect that the change will benefit you and not disadvantage others, although it may require them to work in a different way.

What is the change that you intend to negotiate? (Choose a minor issue for your first attempt)

What are the potential advantages for you, and for others?

What are the potential disadvantages for you, and for others?

EXERCISE 6   Continued.

What facts relate to your case (the full facts about potential winners and losers)?

Who will the change affect, and how will they be affected?

How and where will you put your case?

What is your 'bottom line' – that is, what is the limit or extent of changes you propose that will satisfy your purpose?

What is likely to be the others' 'bottom line'?

Have you other ideas or suggestions to offer that might be used as bargaining tools?

What are your plans for tackling which people, when and where?

FEELING GOOD BY RAISING YOUR SELF-ESTEEM

Even apparently confident people may suffer from low self-esteem. Some people blame the hierarchical training of nurses, in which student nurses were constantly told how low they were in the pecking order, and doctors seemed to be infallible. The personality trait of self-criticism is a strong predictor of whether a health professional will feel stressed, so learning to tolerate failures in yourself is an important target to attain in your fight against stress.

Individuals can deliberately raise their self-esteem by positive tactics and thinking. However, to effect any change you must be prepared to take the risk of failure – success is not automatic. And to ride failures successfully you have to develop a positive approach before you start, so that you can set yourself up to learn from failure rather than being cast down by it.

Below are some positive strategies to raise your self-esteem.

1 Accept that not every attempt to change will be a success.

2 Be prepared to take a risk to effect a change in your life.

3 Try positive visualisation, i.e. imagine yourself successfully managing a forthcoming event or activity about which you are feeling apprehensive.

4 Use positive body language – people will treat you more positively, too.

5 Review and recall past successes and hold them in the forefront of your mind.

6 Learn from any mistakes or failures, and don't dismiss such experiences.

7 Learn to feel comfortable with yourself – physically and mentally.

8 Write your worries down and review them periodically, rather than continually fretting over them.

9 Be aware of your good points, and constantly reinforce them in your thinking.

10 Do the best for yourself and give yourself every opportunity to succeed – don't set yourself up to fail.

EXERCISE 7   Review the state of your self-esteem.

Do you need to concentrate on trying to raise your self-esteem? If so, write down any positive strategies you could adopt to increase your self-esteem. If your self-esteem is pretty good, what can you do to maintain it? What will you do and when?

1

2

3

4

When will you review the outcomes of this exercise?

AVOIDING AGGRESSION AND VIOLENCE AT WORK

The problem of aggression and violence at work is common in the general working population, with around 35 000 people being attacked at work across the UK each year. The British Crime Survey reported that health professionals appear to be at higher risk of work-related violence (including woundings, common assault, robbery and snatch theft) than the general population, with records showing a frequency of 580 incidents per 10 000 nurses and midwives in 1995.[1]

Nurses are particularly vulnerable to aggression and violence. Some nurses have a great deal of daily one-to-one contact with patients who are mentally ill or disturbed, in circumstances where emotions run high and normally sane patients or relatives can suddenly become irrational or aggressive. Practice and community nurses, doctors and other health-care staff who visit patients in their own homes are often unaware of risks to their safety, because their caring nature and their role as the patient's advocate make them relatively unsuspicious of danger.

Even if they have never experienced actual violence themselves, many nurses know of vicious attacks on other doctors and nurses, and have been the victims of verbal abuse and physical threats at some time in their careers. All of this may create an atmosphere of fear about their personal safety on visits to patients' homes.

The best way to reduce stress arising from aggression and violence is to prevent the episode from occurring in the first place. This will include:

- avoiding potentially dangerous situations, especially when on visits to patients' homes

- learning how to defuse tense confrontations

- improving the workplace organisation so that the service provided is efficient

- devising a workplace policy to handle a violent or aggressive incident

- equipping staff with assertiveness and anger management skills

- offering support to staff who have been victims of attack or abuse

- learning from any violent episode, and making changes to avoid a recurrence.

Although nurses have a duty to provide care and uphold patient confidentiality (according to the UKCC Code of Professional Conduct), abuse and violence from a patient cancel this contract. Guidance from the Royal College of Nursing[2,3] advises any nurse who has been seriously assaulted that they have the right to report the incident to the police, thus breaking confidentiality with regard to the name and contact details of the assailant.

Under-reporting of violent episodes is said to be widespread, and people have different perceptions about behaviour which they regard as threatening or offensive. Sometimes nurses, such as those working in Accident and Emergency Units, may tolerate particular patients' rudeness or threats and accept them uncomplainingly as a way of life.

Verbal abuse is thought to be at one end of a continuing spectrum that ends in physical assault. Such episodes should be treated seriously and not dismissed as trivial just because they were not accompanied by physical attack.

⟵――――――――――――――――――――――――――――――⟶

Verbal abuse	Threats/gestures	Physical contact (pushing, etc.)	Attack

Nurse victim(s) of any violent incidents at work should be encouraged to talk about their experiences and be debriefed as soon as possible after the event, or stress will invariably result. A workplace policy should be in existence with which everyone is familiar, to reduce the likelihood of aggression and violence flaring at work, to defuse any such incident effectively, to summon help as necessary, and to counsel and support any victim(s) afterwards.

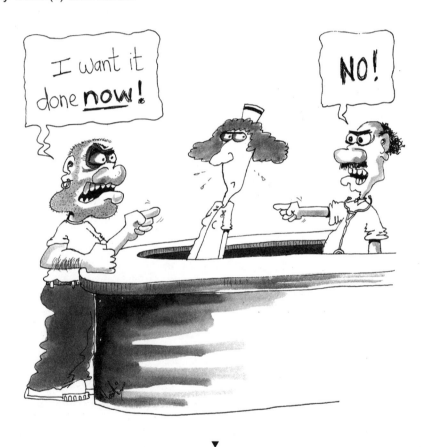

▼

Avoiding aggression.

Avoiding circumstances that lead to aggression and violence

Violent behaviour can flare up unexpectedly even for those working in pleasant middle-class areas. However, being able to recognise early warning signs of aggression and being more aware of risky situations should allow nurses to be better prepared to disarm anger and defuse potentially violent situations.

For nurses, the particular circumstances in which the risks of violence are more likely[4] occur when they are:

- working alone
- working after normal working hours
- travelling to and working in patients' homes
- withholding a service
- exercising authority
- working with people who are emotionally or mentally unstable
- working with people who are under the influence of alcohol or drugs
- working with people under stress.

Sometimes a particular patient may behave well with some of the staff but be aggressive or abusive to others. Whatever action is taken against the patient should have the full backing of all of the managers of the practice or Trust. A distinction must be made between those patients who behave badly of their own volition, and those who are temporarily mentally disturbed, e.g. with a psychosis. Medical or nursing staff who are assaulted by a psychotic patient as part of their illness may rightly be more tolerant and not prosecute him or her, but treat the patient instead.

Self-defence courses may teach new skills which would only be used as a last resort. It is worth carrying out a regular review of potential risks to staff and their personal security, and then instituting any changes that may reduce the risk of violence or aggression at work. Episodes of aggression or violence occurring in the workplace should be reported and incident record forms completed which are examined at least annually, to look for trends and patterns.

Unfortunately, even in reasonably happy workplaces, aggression sometimes erupts between staff. Such incidents usually arise when communication in the team is poor and the management is weak. Interpersonal conflicts can create a lot of passion, and the cause of the dispute needs to be sorted out quickly and resolved before colleagues divide into two factions supporting one party or the other.

How you say things is more important than what you say. Any nurse under threat of violence should try to appear confident and assertive but not aggressive, and they should be aware of the messages given out by their body language from the very first moment that the patient starts to act in an aggressive way. Normally nurses would put patients at their ease in any case. Defusing tension by remaining calm and unhurried is really just an extension of their normal manner.

The value of early counselling after a violent incident has been demonstrated by reducing the amount of sick-leave that a 'victim' takes. There should be someone in the workplace who will take responsibility for listening to and supporting the person who has been attacked or upset by another's aggression. Any post-traumatic stress will be lessened by effective support from others at work, and by the knowledge that the manager will try to change the workplace or organisation in some way so as to reduce the likelihood of a recurrence.

**Key points to consider when trying to minimise the risk
to nursing staff[4]:**

- physical aspects of the workplace

- working patterns and practices

- staffing levels and competence

- staff training in defusing and controlling aggression and violence

- personal, organisational and premises security arrangements

- response strategies, both at the time and afterwards.

Tips for avoiding violence and aggression from patients whilst making home visits

- Don't enter a house without an escort, preferably the police, if you suspect the possibility of violence.

- Stay nearest to the door – leave it open for a speedy escape.

- If you feel insecure, switch your mobile phone on before you enter the house and arrange for someone back at the workplace to listen in while you are inside. They can then summon help quickly if necessary.

- Withdraw quickly at any sign of danger. Don't be brave or foolhardy. If there is a knife about leave if you can.

- Carry your nursing equipment in your pockets or an inconspicuous bag.

- Ask the caller to ensure that there is good lighting from their house, with the upstairs curtains drawn open, to enable you to find it more easily if it is dark.

- Make sure that you have crystal-clear instructions on how to find the house so that you do not have to wander about searching for it. Mark house numbers on your local maps, especially if the numbering is illogical.

- Be polite, courteous and non-aggressive, however frustrated and angry you feel inside.

EXERCISE 8   Review the safety and security arrangements for preventing the likelihood of violence and aggression to nurses and other staff at your workplace, and for handling it as effectively as possible if it does occur.

How does your workplace or organisation measure up? Circle the types of systems or procedures that exist:

Preventive	In response to a violent episode
Staff training	Support
Team approach	Report
Adequate staffing	Analyse
Secure premises	Discuss
Surgery alarms	Change systems
Good environment	Review policy
Good communication	Prosecute
Practice policy	
Planned interventions for different eventualities	
General awareness of danger	
Good organisation	
Culture of concern for staff	

What are the most dangerous situations *for you* at work, and what changes can you make to minimise the likelihood of aggression and violence occurring?

Potentially threatening situations	Intended changes
•	
•	
•	
•	

References

1 Home Office (1996) *British Crime Survey.* Home Office Research and Statistics Directorate, London.

2 Royal College of Nursing (1998) *Dealing with violence against nursing staff.* Royal College of Nursing, London.

3 Royal College of Nursing (1998) *Safer working in the community: a guide for NHS managers and staff on reducing the risks from violence and aggression.* Royal College of Nursing, London.

4 Health Services Advisory Committee (1998) *Violence and aggression in general practice: guidance on assessment and management.* Health and Safety Executive, London.

Other reading

Clarke D (1989) *Stress management: assertion training.* National Extension College, Cambridge.

Cozens J (1991) *OK2 talk feelings.* BBC Books, London.

Davies P (1996) *Personal power: how to become more assertive and successful at work.* Piatkus, London.

Denny R (1997) *Succeed for yourself: unlock your potential for success and happiness.* Kogan Page, London.

Jeffers S (1987) *Feel the fear and do it anyway.* Rider, London.

Palladino C (1994) *Developing self-esteem.* Crisp Publications, California.

Audio-cassettes

Wendy Lloyd Audio Productions Ltd. For the twin tapes of 'Feeling good': 30 Guffitts Rake, Meols, Wirral L47 7AD. Tel: 0151 632 0662.

Sources of information

Victim Support National Office: Cranmer House, 39 Brixton Road, London SW9 6DZ. Tel: 0171 735 9166.

Health and Safety Executive: Rose Court, Magdalen House, 2 Southwark Bridge Road, London SE1 9HS. Tel: 0171 717 6000.

MODULE 4
Defining time management

AIMS

The aims of Module 4 are:

1 To increase nurses' repertoire of ways to practise time management.

2 To help nurses to review their priorities and reallocate the relative proportions of their time spent on different activities accordingly.

3 To engage nurses in making action plans to improve their time management.

CONTENTS

The total time needed to work through this module will depend on the amount of time you spend reflecting on how the information in the module applies to you, before completing the exercises. The total time that might be spent on this module is 12 hours (including time for reading, thinking, and undertaking the daily activities logs and the significant event analyses).

Below are the comments that some participants made about the benefits they had gained from undertaking previous *Survival Skills* programmes.

About the time-management programme:

'I had to find time to complete this programme, but it was worthwhile and very educational.'

'It made me take time to appraise my situation and endeavour to improve the quality of my life.'

'Lack of a time limit means that the programme can be lived with over a period of time.'

'It forced me to make time to think around the subjects involved.'

About applying time-management skills:

'It enabled me to use time at work effectively.'

'It has made me make changes.'

'It has helped me to organise myself better.'

'I have a better insight into how I get distracted by other members of staff and unimportant jobs at work.'

'I have learnt to manage my time working at the practice better. For instance, I have changed the length of time for which appointments are booked, which I've been thinking about for years.'

'I get more done by prioritising the jobs better. I even go home on time these days.'

KEY PRINCIPLES OF TIME MANAGEMENT

This workbook is all about being smarter about getting through your work. A certain degree of time pressure is probably necessary for you to maintain your interest and momentum in getting a job done. However, too much pressure could tip you over the peak of your performance, so that you are less efficient and your work suffers as you become less effective.

Nurses are conditioned by their training and work to feel that they must cope, whatever the time pressures. They feel that patients must not suffer, whatever the costs to the nurses themselves. However, there are limits to nurses' tolerance, and if too much pressure is exerted in this way for too long a time, some nurses may end up feeling 'burnt out' and consider leaving their job or profession. So you must learn to control the demands on your time, before any excessive pressures affect you and your performance adversely.

One of the most common sources of stress for nurses is time pressure. The key to good time management is to:

- balance your work and leisure time
- prioritise how you spend your time – do not allow yourself or others to waste it
- control interruptions
- include sufficient time for thinking, doing, meeting, developing and learning in your working day
- allow sufficient time for the unexpected
- delegate work whenever it is appropriate to do so, at work and at home
- try only to accept delegated work without further training if you have the necessary skills, time and experience
- get on with essential tasks and do not procrastinate
- be assertive – learn to say 'no' often enough to unnecessary work or taking on other people's jobs and tasks
- make effective decisions, and don't look back
- put past mistakes behind you – do not ruminate over them
- review significant problems and learn to manage time better in order to avoid those problems in future by making realistic action plans.

Balance your work and leisure time successfully

One of the secrets of a happy life is to get the balance of stress right. Some stress is healthy, too much is not! The object is to achieve just enough stress to encourage optimum performance and enjoyment, but not so much as to make work seem an endless grind and impair performance.

One of the ways to reduce stress is to timetable enough free time during your day to have space for rest and relaxation to counteract the stresses and strains of your working life.

Try and complete work activities within your normal working shifts, so that you have enough time for non-work-related activities in your life. If you do not allow sufficient time for leisure, you will not have the opportunity for personal growth outside work and will probably become stale. Every so often, you might set a target to learn or improve at something outside work or take active measures to nurture your relationship with your spouse, family and friends, e.g. by sharing a new hobby.

The best options are solutions that make regular time and space for yourself for fun, relaxation, hobbies and enjoying simple pleasures throughout your life as a *stress-proofing* measure. Don't suddenly try and adopt these methods to beat stress at one particular time in your working life, when you are already below par. One of the best ways to monitor whether you are managing to protect enough time for yourself is to keep a daily log of activities for a week or so. At a recent clinical update meeting, the lecturer asked the nurses in the audience to be honest and indicate how much time they had spent in the previous week pursuing an activity that was for *their own* enjoyment. Only a quarter of the audience could say that they had done this, which was a sad state of affairs.

EXERCISE 1   Keep a log of daily activities for a week.

Photocopy the daily log below and record all your activities each day for a week, including an off-duty period if possible. Sort the activities into three separate columns:

- *personal needs*, including shopping, sleeping, domestic chores, bodily needs, etc.

- *work,* including reading work-related books, reports and papers

- *leisure,* including sport, relaxation, reading, music, etc.

Work out totals for the types of activities for each day. Compare your daily recordings with the Health Education Authority's recommendations for a healthy lifestyle by grouping your activities into the same categories:

- 45–55% on personal needs

- 25–30% on work

- 20–25% on leisure.

When the work component increases above 25%, it is usually the leisure proportion of the day that is reduced.

Daily log of activities

TIME SPENT ON ACTIVITY
(To nearest quarter of an hour):

Personal needs (*shopping, washing, domestic chores, sleeping*)		Work		Leisure	
Activity	Time spent	Activity	Time spent	Activity	Time spent
	Total for day:		Total for day:		Total for day:

Defining time management

EXERCISE 1   Continued.

Review of log of several days' activities

How do your totals compare with the Health Education Authority's guidelines? Enter your totals here:

- Personal needs:

- Work:

- Leisure:

Can you note any trends or patterns of activities, e.g. staying late at work, catching up on paperwork at home, from your daily time logs?

Were you generally in control of the time spent on different activities in your days, or did events control you? (*Yes, I was in control /No, events controlled me*)

For what proportion of your days' timetables were your activities fixed (e.g. management or case meetings or clinics)? Write in how many hours are generally under your control each day where activities might be rescheduled in another way.

- Number of hours at work under your control:

- Number of hours outside work under your control:

What were the biggest time-wasters for you?

- At work:

- Outside work:

How much of your leisure time was spent doing what you wanted to do?

Were there any surprises arising from the daily time logs?

Do you need to make changes in your life in order to create more protected time for yourself (and your family)? What do you intend to do, and when?

Intend to	Start date
1	
2	
3	
4	
5	

Prioritise your time: do not allow yourself or others to waste it

The first step is to be clear about your goals in your work and home life, and leisure. How you allot your time will look very different if your main goal is to be a great golfer, to learn a new skill such as aromatherapy or nurse prescribing, or to spend as much time as possible with your family. Plan your goals in association with whoever else they affect, and make sure that if you have more than one goal they do not conflict with each other.

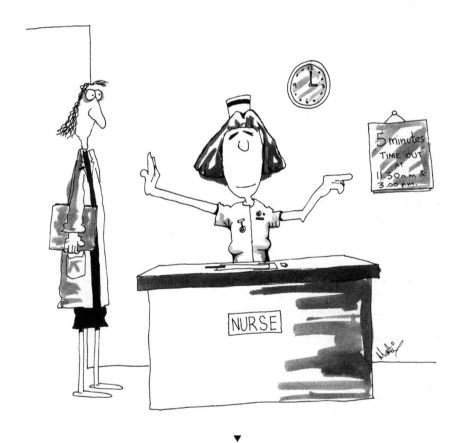

▼
Prioritise your time.

EXERCISE 2   Plan to achieve your goals.

1 *What goals do you want to achieve in the context of work?*

During this next month?

During this coming year?

2 *What goals do you want to achieve outside work?*

During this next month?

During this coming year?

Set out your strategies for how you will achieve your goals. What is hindering you? What will help you?

3 *What steps could you take to achieve your work goals (speak to your manager, plan for your next performance appraisal, training, resources, set aside time, tasks, etc.)?*

In the next month?

In the next year?

4 *What steps could you take to achieve your goals outside work (find out about opportunities for training, set aside time, tasks, etc.)?*

In the next month?

In the next year?

Now that you have clarified your goals and have set out your strategies to achieve those goals, you need to structure sufficient time around those priorities. Look back at the results of your week of logging time spent on daily activities, and map out the activities and tasks that are essential at work and at home. Programme your priority activities in, either as a paper exercise or by thinking it through and resolving a new schedule.

When an activity arises and you have a choice about taking it on or not, match it against your goals. If it takes you further away from your goals, then refuse to take it on, but if it brings you closer to achieving your goals, consider if you have time to fit it in. Be firm with yourself and do not agree to do it just because you like the person who is asking you and want to please him or her. Guard against being distracted from your overall objectives by the hurly-burly of work.

Make sure that you spend your quality time doing the most important or complex jobs. It is too easy to focus on completing small unimportant tasks and put off tackling the big ones, which just hang over you and make you feel guilty about leaving them unattended.

A high-priority task has to be done, a medium-priority job may be delegated, and a low-priority task should only be done if you have no medium- or high-priority tasks waiting, or you are too jaded to tackle them.

EXERCISE 3   Work out a timetabled programme to achieve the goals that you have just set out for achieving at work and outside work.

Goal 1   The work goal that you want to achieve by the end of a month.

When and how? Where and what will you do?

How will you know that you have achieved your goal?

Goal 2   The work goal that you want to achieve by the end of the year.

When and how? Where and what will you do?

How will you know that you have achieved your goal?

Defining time management   **95**

Goal 3   The goal for outside work that you want to achieve by the
          end of a month.

When and how? Where and what will you do?

How will you know that you have achieved your goal?

Goal 4   The goal for outside work that you want to achieve by the
          end of a year.

When and how? Where and what will you do?

How will you know that you have achieved your goal?

Control interruptions

Interruptions are one of the biggest timewasters, especially if someone else
could have handled the problem or taken the message, or no action was
required. Even if an interruption is necessary, it may occur at the wrong
time, wrecking your concentration or train of thought. Agree upon rules in
your workplace about who may be interrupted and when. Work out a
system (and keep to it!) with your colleagues and manager at work for
letting others know when you are not to be disturbed and are spending
quality time on priority tasks, and when you are available to deal with the
queries that have built up while you were occupied. Keep focused on your
priorities, and don't allow others to engage you in idle chatter when you are
intent on work. Nurses' concentration may be continually distracted, for
example, if other staff constantly invade the treatment room to fetch

---

Defining time management

equipment while they are in the middle of treating patients. Nurses working in the community may feel frustrated and time-pressured if they have to keep breaking off from their rounds and journeying back to base for briefing meetings held at inconvenient times, or when it was not necessary to deliver the briefing in person.

You could get into the habit of regarding minutes or hours as costed time. Think of how much some of the activities on which you spend time are worth, and whether different activities are of equal worth.

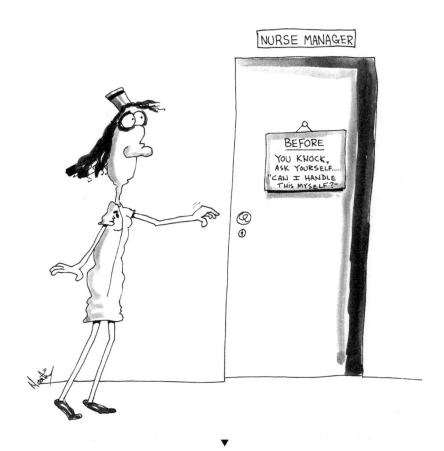

▼
Control interruptions.

EXERCISE 4   Tackle interruptions.

Which interruptions plague you most? Are they necessary? You should be able to think of ways to minimise them effectively.

- Write down the most *frequent* interruption you receive at work.

- How could you minimise this kind of interruption occurring and/or its effect on you?

- So what changes will you make now?

- Write down what is the most *annoying* interruption at work.

- How can you minimise this kind of interruption occurring and/or its effect on you?

- So what changes will you make now?

Include sufficient time for thinking, doing, meeting, developing and learning

You need to be fresh and creative in order to stay on top of the demands made on you as a nurse and remain productive. You can only manage this in the longer term if you have the right mix of stimulating work, personal and professional development and networking regularly timetabled into your daily schedule. Persistent overwork will be counterproductive and will become a negative stress which may lead to you becoming less effective.

You will achieve more in designated sessions of quiet, uninterrupted time than in a longer allocated period of time broken up by various activities. This is the time for planning, writing reports or analysing progress.

Try to allow at least 10% of your time for dealing with unexpected tasks. Looking after patients invariably means that you will have unexpected work to do. In the unlikely event that everything goes smoothly and you do not need the extra time, it will be a bonus to have that additional space to catch up on the backlog of paperwork, or simply to spend a little more time talking to patients about how they are feeling.

You will have your own preference for thinking time, which to some extent will depend on your personality. Extroverts will be revitalised by brainstorming and discussions with a group of others, while those who are more introverted will prefer protected space in which to reflect and read. Whichever of these you prefer, make sure that you get enough of it to replenish your creativity and enthusiasm. Some nurses join local groups with like-minded colleagues that provide a mix of support, education and social activities. More nurses are joining in the trend to be part of a clinical supervision group. Learning sets are springing up, offering development and support in small groups of peers of nurses and/or others from different health disciplines. You might benefit from finding a buddy who is a nurse like you, to listen to each other and exchange ideas and support through regular meetings.

EXERCISE 5 Consider whether you are spending enough time on personal and professional development.

• When did you last have enough space in your working day to *think* about anything developmental?

• Are you satisfied with the amount of time you have for personal and professional development?

• If you are dissatisfied, how can you clear space in your working day to attend an educational event on something you want to learn?

• When will you approach your colleagues and manager about timetabling this in?

• What could you realistically stop doing in order to accommodate this developmental time for yourself?

• What arrangements could be made to protect this self-development time – for example, could other nursing colleagues cover for you?

Delegate whatever and however you can; try only to accept delegated work without further training if you have the necessary skills, time and experience

Nurses are usually on the receiving end of delegated work, certainly more often than they are on the delegating side. If you are in a position to delegate work and responsibilities, decide what only *you* can do, and delegate as much as possible of the rest to others. It is important to reduce duplication as much as possible so that work and initiatives are co-ordinated over different disciplines wherever this is feasible and, for example, social workers, district nurses and practice nurses are not doing similar work with the same patients in parallel or in duplicate.

If you are usually on the receiving end of delegated work, try to make sure that you understand what is required, and that you have the necessary time, skills and experience, before agreeing or acquiescing to taking on the new work. Communication among and between medical and nursing staff is often poor if everyone is in a rush. There is great potential for time-wasting if you try to carry out delegated work when you don't know what is required or how to set about doing it. If you don't have the time or skills for the additional work, try and negotiate how you will obtain the necessary training and when you will do the work in your most assertive manner.

You should consider delegation not just at work, but also at home. If you find it difficult to relinquish control, and like to be seen as achieving in all spheres of your life – super-nurse, super-homemaker, super-parent, super-spouse, etc., you may need convincing that it is perfectly acceptable to minimise the chores at home when you are so busy at work. If you can afford it, employing domestic or gardening help is one of the most effective ways of instantly obtaining more quality time at home. If you cannot afford it, you will have to recruit all of the family to help on a fair rota system, rather than trying to do most of the chores by yourself.

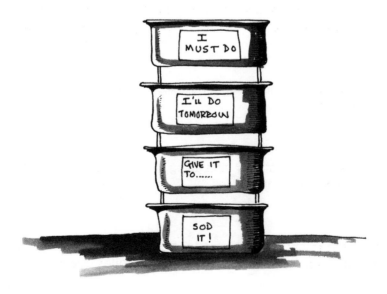

▼

Prioritise and delegate.

EXERCISE 6   Consider whether you are delegating work effectively and appropriately.

At work:

• Could you delegate work more than you do?

• To whom could you delegate more work?

• What is stopping you from delegating more work (for example, too few clerical staff)?

• What arrangements will you make to delegate more work? When and how?

• How often are you on the receiving end of work that is inappropriately delegated to you?

• How will you react next time someone tries to delegate work to you without there being any extra time in which to do it?

• How will you react next time someone tries to delegate work to you without you having what you consider to be the necessary skills or experience to undertake that work?

At home:

• Could you delegate work more than you do?

• To whom could you delegate more work?

• What is stopping you from delegating more work?

• What arrangements will you make to delegate more work? When and how?

Don't procrastinate: get on with essential tasks

So what are you waiting for? Distasteful or complicated tasks are the ones people procrastinate over. However, if it is an essential or important task you will have to do it sometime, and you will only feel guilty about putting it off. If you procrastinate for too long, the job will be even more difficult, as you will forget your previous ideas or what the instructions were. If you train yourself to do the least wanted task first, you can reward yourself with a more pleasing job or even free time.

Wait until you have time to complete one stage or the whole of a job. Don't pick up a piece of paper and half read it, decide that it is too difficult to tackle or that you haven't enough time, and put it down again. You will have wasted that time deciding to put it off, and if you are in this procrastinating state of mind you may also welcome unnecessary interruptions and compound the time-wasting further. Try to get yourself geared up for the job and launch into it.

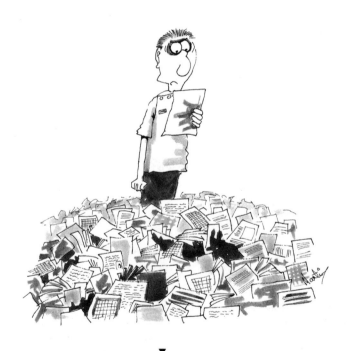

▼
Don't procrastinate.

EXERCISE 7   Are you procrastinating too often?

- What task or job are you most likely to procrastinate over?

- How might you force yourself to get on and do the job?

- What reward or incentive might you use to discourage yourself from procrastinating?

- So what is your plan to avoid procrastinating over this task in future?

Control your work flow

As well as using the control techniques described above, you should review the flow of your work to match your capacity. You are more likely to be most productive with a steady flow of work, rather than arranging your day as a pressure/slack/pressure sandwich. If you work in a general practice, the surgery times may mean that there is 'dead time' in the middle of the day when you are less productive because the pressure is off and you waste time by taking longer to do small tasks, only to find that you invariably finish work late after a pressured evening surgery. If that is the case, you will have to find ways as a practice to change the work flow in the system to suit you better, by changing booking times, or moving evening meetings to earlier slots in the day, etc. If you work in a hospital setting, you might find that the work flow is uneven if you work in out-patient clinics when the ambulance transport suddenly delivers shoals of patients to the clinics, or when a series of emergencies are admitted to the wards. Again, you will have to organise yourselves as a team to make sure that as many non-urgent tasks as possible are completed during quieter periods to keep up a steady work flow.

Concentrate on one task at a time. Complete it and either move on to another job or take a short break to refresh yourself and clear your mind ready to start again. Don't move from one task to another or you will waste effort, having to start thinking about the topic all over again each time you take it up.

If you are swamped by work you will be less efficient and more forgetful, which may create even more time pressure if you have to put right the problem caused by your forgetting something or missing an appointment. You are likely to be more efficient if you group small, similar tasks together, such as returning telephone calls. Always have one or two small jobs put by or carried with you, so that if you are kept waiting you can get on with those tasks and not waste time. Maintain control of your paperwork. Don't let it build up so that you feel overwhelmed or you will either put off tackling it altogether, or work more slowly because the enormity of the task depresses you.

Limit the time you spend on the telephone. If you measure how long you talk for the next few times you are on the telephone you will probably be surprised by how many minutes the calls last for. Listen to yourself, and you may find that much of the time is spent on pleasantries or repeating what you have already said.

EXERCISE 8   Are you in control of your work, or does it control you?

- Do you control your work as much as possible, or do you let the work control you?

- What changes could you make to control the flow of your work, in line with the ideas described above?

- When will you start?

- What will you do?

- Will these changes have any knock-on effects on you or anyone else?

Be assertive: say 'No' to unnecessary work or other people's jobs and tasks

The biggest challenge is to be assertive with yourself so that you don't agree to take on additional tasks that are not essential for you to do, or that fall outside your own priority areas. If you are not careful you may be so busy helping others that you do not get your own work done.

Module 3 on dealing with assertiveness techniques will give you more detailed help.

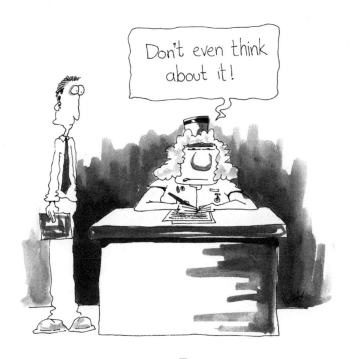

▼

Say 'No'.

Make effective decisions

Be decisive and finish jobs in hand. Collect information about a problem or choice, weigh up the pros and cons and make a decision. Once you have made that decision, look forward and make plans for the future – don't look backwards and frame regrets. Below are some tips on making effective decisions.

- There are always other options – find out what they are.

- Gather ideas and evidence from other people or a range of sources – do not be confined only to the options you already know about.

- Base your analyses and decision on reliable objective evidence or observations, and not on 'guesstimates'.

- Think through the implications of your decision by considering the possible consequences before choosing which options to take.

- Information is about feelings as well as facts – how the situation really is and how people feel about it.

- Your personality and beliefs will affect your decision-making process.

- Don't accept other people's perceptions of reality – look and think for yourself.

- Be honest with yourself and others, and keep your integrity. The best decisions are based on truth and not illusions.

- Effective decisions are based on reality and not hope.

- Probing questions help to distinguish between illusion and reality.

- Simple decisions are usually best, and are often obvious in retrospect.

- Fear gets in the way of making realistic assessments of the options.

- Don't make decisions because you are frightened of something, but because you are enthusiastic about the expected outcomes.

The more aware you are of your own character, the better you will understand how you make decisions. How you feel about how you make a decision often forecasts the results. If you feel good about a decision, the outcome is usually a success.

EXERCISE 9   Look at how good you are at making effective decisions.

- How good do you think you are in general at making effective decisions?

- What is stopping you from being more decisive?

- How often do you regret a decision that you have made? (*Often/seldom/never*)

- How often do you ruminate over decisions, thinking over and over again whether you did the right thing? (*Often/seldom/never*)

Describe an important decision that you have to make now or in the near future.

- What are the options?

- What are the circumstances or potential advantages of your preferred option?

- What are the circumstances or potential disadvantages of your preferred option?

- What other information do you need to obtain before making your decision?

- How sure are you that you have all the information possible, and have thought through the consequences of your decision both for yourself and for other people?

- If you have decided not to make any decision in the short term, when will you review the situation?

- To what extent do you expect your decision to be a positive choice rather than one that simply makes the best of things?

- Is there any other way that you could be more effective about making this decision?

EXERCISE 10   Which time-management techniques have worked for you in the past?

Which do you still use? Tick which principles work for you in the table below.

Time-management principles	Tried in the past	Use now	Work for you
Keep a time log of activities and review it			
Write down tasks – prioritise them and make an action plan			
Reduce unnecessary activities			
Get work in perspective and limit time spent			
Delegate appropriately			
Go on a formal course – time for reflection			
Whenever possible, handle each piece of paper only once – deal with it straight away			
Say 'No' to extra work			
Don't take on other people's jobs/tasks			
Set aside 'thinking' time			
Allow time for unexpected tasks (10%?)			
Be brief on the telephone			
Tackle one task at a time – finish it			
Prepare for meetings to be effective			
Listen carefully and so act correctly first time			
Don't procrastinate – do it now			
Do difficult tasks when you are most alert			

MAKING ACTION PLANS TO MANAGE YOUR TIME BETTER

Undertaking a significant event analysis of a frequently occurring time-management problem or an unexpected crisis is a good way to work out the basis for a timetabled action programme to manage time better for you either as an individual or as a team.

Read through the example below, and then work through two significant event analyses yourself – of you as an individual, and as one of your workplace team, unless you can persuade all the rest of your team to join in, too, in which case you should include everybody as in the example described below.

Example of introducing an intervention to reduce the stress of telephone interruptions to a nurse during a surgery or clinic in a general practice, community clinic or hospital setting

Stage 1

Time stress topic chosen: *reducing telephone interruptions in clinic.* This is an intervention concerned with preventing time stresses on the individual nurse. Reason for choice: *because telephone interruptions are a frequent cause of stress to nurses.*

In this example it seemed as if such interruptions occurred at least 10 times every clinic before the nurse set about recording whether this was really the case.

Stage 2

The standard might be as follows. Telephone interruptions during clinics will only be permitted if a patient telephones with an emergency problem, or if a senior nurse, manager or doctor telephones and cannot be contacted easily after the clinic has finished. The standard should be set by the manager and all of the clinical and administrative staff in the workplace.

Stage 3

Everyone agrees to the plan. No new skill training is needed. The new arrangements will include a well-advertised 30-minute time slot after the clinic when patients and others can speak directly to the nurse and other staff.

Their action plan is as follows.

1 The workplace team agree standards – no telephone interruptions other than from medical and nursing colleagues who will not be easily contactable later on, and from patients with emergency requests.

Defining time management

2 Seek agreement for proposed standards with the appropriate manager and senior colleagues.

3 Nominate a project leader (a senior nurse in this case).

4 Decide how the new system of 30-minute telephone contact time at the end of clinics will operate (workplace staff).

5 Inform receptionists and all staff of the start date for the new system of putting telephone calls straight through to the nurse.

6 Put a notice up in the waiting-room to inform patients that the trial system is running, and send memos to others in the organisation who are likely to be affected.

7 Expected outcome(s):

- Advantage: the nurse will feel less time-pressured during patient consultations in the surgery or clinic.

- Disadvantage: the nurse may be delayed after the end of the clinic or surgery, waiting for the 30-minute telephone contact time to expire.

Stage 4

Prepare data-recording forms, photocopy them and distribute.

Stage 5

Collect baseline information. All nurses are to record how many times they are interrupted during each surgery or clinic for one week before the new system is introduced. The recording should also note how many of the interruptions are from medical colleagues or patients with urgent or emergency requests.

Stage 6

Start the new system of telephone contact time. During the week after the new system is introduced, all nurses are to record the number of and reason(s) for telephone interruptions during surgeries or clinics and throughout telephone contact times. (See example of data collection form overleaf for one nurse recording the number of and reasons for telephone interruptions per weekday.)

Stage 7

The project leader compares the nurses' results as an aggregated anonymised comparison of the week's recordings of numbers of and reasons for telephone contacts after the new system was introduced compared to:

1 before the new system was introduced

2 the standards set at the beginning of the project.

Stage 8

Feedback of these comparative results is given to nurses and other staff. (In this case, performance was better than before the new system was introduced, when there were as many as 10 telephone interruptions per surgery, but not as good as the agreed standards, as there were still some telephone calls that were not emergency requests or from medical or nursing colleagues, that were being put through to the nurse according to the example data-collection recording chart shown below.)

Review of outcomes:

1 Advantages of new system:

- Nurses feel less time-pressured and consequently feel less stressed without so many interruptions.

- Nurses are able to concentrate on seeing patients without being distracted by interruptions.

- Nurses are less likely to make mistakes during clinics and surgeries (e.g. treatment errors, forgetting to call patients, mistakes on test forms) with fewer interruptions occurring.

2 Disadvantages of new system:

- Patients may be unaware of the new system and so telephone in twice as much – first to try to speak to the nurse during surgery or clinic times, and secondly to make the postponed call.

- Nurses may be delayed leaving the surgery or clinic if they are waiting for the designated telephone contact time to expire.

- Patients may feel dissatisfied with the service if their previously easy access to the nurse is restricted.

Stage 9

Monitoring is carried out one month later by nurses recording the number and type of interruptions for a few days, especially to ensure that patients are not abusing the easy telephone access to nurses at the end of the surgery or clinic by telephoning to discuss trivial matters.

Example of daily data collection form

Number of and reasons for interruptions one week after new system has been introduced

Weekday: (Monday/Tuesday/Wednesday/Thursday/Friday)

Morning surgery/clinic:	3
Afternoon surgery/clinic:	Not in surgery
Evening surgery/clinic:	2
Type of telephone call:	
• medical/nursing colleague	1
• emergency request from patient	1
• not medical colleague or emergency	3

EXERCISE 11 Undertake an analysis of a significant event involving a time-management problem at work for you as an individual.

Focus on analysing the significant event from the perspective of preventing the time-management problem for you as an *individual*. Your aim will be to reduce or change the nature of the time stressor – to remove the 'hazard' or reduce the frequency/extent of the time stressor. If prevention is impossible, a secondary approach would be to alter the ways in which you as an individual respond to the time stressor, or to improve your ability to recognise and deal with time-related problems as they arise.

Stage 1

Write down a factual account of the time-pressured situation you have chosen – who was involved, what time of day, and what task or activity you were engaged in. The situation should be a frequent source of time stress, an important cause of time stress, or an infrequent event which, when it occurs, has far-reaching effects, or a time stress which is costly in terms of time or resources. It must be a realistic choice, i.e. a cause of time stress which you can reasonably expect to be able to reduce.

Stage 2

Set a 'standard' or a sensible target to aim at that is a recognisable measurement of an acceptable reduction in the time stress that you hope to achieve after you have introduced a new system to reduce the cause of that stress. You may need to carry out a baseline data collection first to provide sufficient information to set the standard if there is no obvious reference point. Record the effects of this cause of time stress on you.

Stage 3

Write out a plan to reduce the time pressure, including the expected outcomes and the anticipated benefits and disadvantages. Discuss your proposal with everyone else involved, at home and at work. Obtain the agreement of anyone who may be concerned by the proposed changes to your set standard(s) and your proposed intervention(s). Amend your plans in the light of others' comments.

EXERCISE 11   Continued.

Stage 4

Prepare to carry out your plan. This will include obtaining or buying any extra equipment, training yourself or others (one of the clerical staff to do more of the paperwork?) if new skills are required, applying for extra staff time or making other resource or organisational arrangements.

Stage 5

Record current performance as a baseline before making any changes. The data collection form on page 115 may be helpful at this stage. Photocopy it and fill in your own row and column headings as appropriate for your project.

Stage 6

Introduce and carry out the intervention, e.g. starting the new system or beginning to use new equipment. Record the new performance measures.

Stage 7

Compare the new performance with the old performance, and with pre-set standards. Has the agreed standard been reached?

Stage 8

Feed back information about the comparison of performance (i.e. Stage 6 results), outcomes of intervention(s) and the improvements or changes to those involved in or affected by the project. Discuss this as a work team and agree and make further changes if the standards have still not been met. Arrange further training, etc., if current skills are still inadequate.

Stage 9

Monitor performance 3 to 6 months later. Reinforce interventions and/or changes, etc., as necessary.

EXERCISE 12   Undertake an analysis of a significant event involving a time-management problem for your workplace team.

For this exercise, focus on analysing the significant event from the perspective of preventing that time-management problem in your workplace team by reducing or changing the nature of the time pressure – removing the 'hazard' or reducing the frequency or extent of the time stressor. If prevention is impossible, a secondary approach would be to alter the ways in which you as a work team respond to the time stressor, or to improve your ability to recognise and deal with time-related problems as they arise.

Stage 1

Write down a factual account of the circumstances of the time-pressured situation you have chosen to review – who is generally involved, the time of day, and the task or activity concerned. The situation should be a frequent source of time stress, an important cause of time stress, or an infrequent event which, when it occurs, has far-reaching effects, or a time stress which is costly in terms of time or resources. It must be a realistic choice, i.e. a cause of time stress which your workplace team can reasonably expect to be able to reduce.

Stage 2

Set a 'standard' agreed with others from your workplace or from published literature, or pick a sensible target to aim at that is a recognisable measurement of an acceptable reduction in the time pressure that you hope to achieve after you have introduced a new system to reduce the cause of that stress. You may need to carry out a baseline data collection first to provide sufficient information to set the standard if there is no obvious reference point.

Write down the effects of time pressure on the participants in the crisis or stressful situation you have chosen.

Stage 3

Write out a plan to reduce the time pressure, including the expected outcomes and the anticipated benefits and disadvantages. Discuss and agree the proposal for change with everyone else involved at work. Obtain the agreement of anyone who may be concerned by the proposed changes to your set standard(s) and your proposed intervention(s). Amend your plans in the light of others' comments.

Stage 4

Prepare to carry out your plan with your workplace team. This will include obtaining or buying any extra equipment, training yourself or others if new skills are required, applying for extra staff time, or making other resource or organisational arrangements.

EXERCISE 12   Continued.

Stage 5

Record your team's current performance as a baseline before making any changes. The data collection form below may be helpful at this stage. Photocopy it and fill in your own row and column headings as appropriate for your project.

Stage 6

Introduce and carry out the intervention, e.g. a new system or using new equipment. Measure your new performance.

Stage 7

Compare your team's new performance with their old performance, and with pre-set standards. Has the agreed standard been reached?

Stage 8

Feed back information about the comparison of your performance (i.e. Stage 6 results), the outcomes of the intervention(s) and the improvements or changes to those involved in or affected by the project. Discuss this as a work team and agree and make further changes if the standards have still not been met. Arrange further training, etc., if current skills still seem to be inadequate.

Stage 9

Monitor your team's performance 3 to 6 months later. Reinforce the interventions and/or changes as necessary.

Data Collection Form

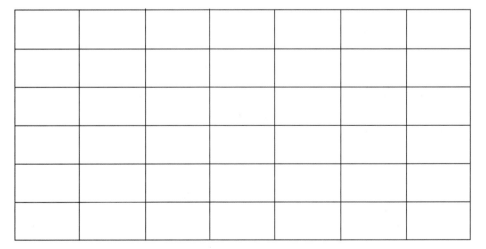

And finally:

EXERCISE 13   Complete a personal contract.

Specify three ways in which you intend to manage time more effectively in future:

What are the obstacles to be overcome? What may stop you acting to manage time more effectively?

What will you do and when will you start?

	Intended action	Start date
1		
2		
3		

Further reading

Clarke D (1989) *Stress management: time management section*. National Extension College, Cambridge.

Garratt S (1985) *Manage your time*. Fontana, London.

MODULE 5
Enhancing job satisfaction

AIMS

The aims of Module 5 are:

1 To increase awareness of the ingredients of job satisfaction among nurses.

2 To engage readers in making plans actively to promote job satisfaction.

3 To encourage a more positive outlook on working as a nurse.

CONTENTS

Developing a positive attitude to your working life

Exercise 17: Identify some positive features of your working and home lives (time to be taken = 20 mins).

Establishing a network of relationships with other colleagues

Exercise 18: Compare your circumstances and workplace with those of other nurses who are satisfied with their jobs (time to be taken = 60 mins).

The total time needed to work through the module might be about 6 hours, depending on the amount of time you spend reflecting on how the information in the module applies to you, before completing the exercises.

Below are the comments of some participants who have used the material in this Module about job satisfaction and their work experiences.

'The course has developed my skills. It has allowed me to appreciate and enjoy aspects of practice which I had overlooked before.'

'I've shifted towards finding time for my own interests instead of those of my family, and this has given me increased satisfaction.'

'It was good to remember my reasons for being a nurse in the first place – good to be reminded of advantages.'

'I'll look to expand my social activities rather than just work.'

'The course is better than classroom teaching because it is reflective.'

'The programme makes you think about your life.'

'The material has given me a greater understanding of my work/family life.'

'Reflecting on my professional development has helped me to get more insight into my strengths and weaknesses.'

'As I listened to other colleagues' views about job satisfaction, the more I came to the conclusion that I need to be in control, instead of allowing other factors, including people, to shape things for me.'

'When I first started my job, I had very little responsibility. I didn't know what was expected of me. I used to go home saying to my husband, if it carries on like this, I'll quit. He said, "Why don't you talk to someone?" So I went to see my manager. We had a long chat about my work. She listened a lot and for that I was grateful. I thought she'd just dismiss me and nothing would come of it. But give her credit, she started giving me more responsibility. Now I feel a new person. I feel I'm doing my part for the team. I feel valued. I feel I can do things for patients and students. Now I'm very satisfied with my work and this programme has encouraged me even more.'

'I find the constant change and uncertainty very demoralising. Health visiting seems to have no future and no direction. Given a chance I will probably leave it.' (Trust-employed health visitor)[1]

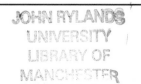

The most important reasons for choosing nursing as a career are said to be 'helping' and 'job satisfaction'.[2] One study of schoolchildren found that pupils aged 10, 15 and 17 years said that they wanted to become a nurse because they 'want to help people to get better'.[3]

CHECKING OUT JOB SATISFACTION

Studies of the general public show that many workers rate job satisfaction and opportunities for learning and personal and professional development more highly than job security or level of earnings. Job satisfaction helps to 'stress-proof' a person and protect them against stress resulting from excessive demands at work. If a person is satisfied by and interested in their job, their motivation will help to keep up standards of performance and the quality of their work despite the pressures of work.

One of the best ways to 'stress-proof' yourself against the pressures of a job is to explore and expand the factors that give you most job satisfaction. If you enjoy your job as a nurse, whether in management, practice or education, and you feel in control of your everyday work and find many aspects of the job satisfying, this will minimise the effects of the parts of the job that you find more stressful.

What about job satisfaction in nursing?

During the early part of 1999 the media focused on the plight of the NHS when there were too many emergency admissions for the number of staff on duty to cope with. In some hospital Trusts staff had to give up their holidays and return to work in order to cope with the crisis created by the unusually high number of admissions. The shortage of nurses was one of the many reasons given to explain the crisis, resulting from difficulties in recruitment and retention of nurses. Not as many people seem to be entering the profession as are leaving the service. Low pay is thought to be one reason why people are leaving the nursing profession or choosing not to enter it. One in seven trainee nurses does not seek registration according to a recent article, and about one-third of student nurses drop out during their training.[4] Thus job satisfaction would seem to be a key factor to explore in this Module, in order to encourage more people to enrol for and complete training as a nurse, and to stay in practice once they are qualified.

In nursing, if you are a relatively junior member of staff or a student, your degree of job satisfaction may be dependent on the way in which senior colleagues treat you. You are more likely to be happy and confident at work if, when a task is delegated, you are given clear instructions, adequate time to do it and help and support throughout the procedure. You will feel that you are being treated as an individual whose needs are being considered. Your self-esteem will be boosted if, when you have completed your task successfully, you are given appropriate feedback[2] and are praised and regarded as a valued member of the team. A study that considered the psychological profiles of nurses found that 'self-esteem' and a 'need to be needed' were crucial for nurses to cope with the job of nursing.[3]

Being a junior member of a team can have its disadvantages as well if students or juniors come to rely on tasks being delegated with full support, so that they have to take minimal responsibility for decision-making and have little control over their work situations. Delegation can reduce a person's autonomy to decide and to establish priorities.[5] In this situation, qualified staff may feel that they are not being given the opportunity to develop. If such a situation persists, it can lead to a great deal of unhappiness and dissatisfaction at work. For example, you may not be in a position to choose when you can have your days off, unless you request them in advance and the staffing situation allows it. Or you may have no control over when you do shift work or when you take holidays. Policies may change and you may find yourself having little leeway in accommodating the needs of your personal circumstances.

Senior staff are in a different position and have relative autonomy. They are mainly in control of how they allocate their time so long as the job is well done, and they are able to deploy resources as they see fit. They not only exert a lot of influence through management, but they are also more likely to achieve their planned goals, because of their position. When people's personal needs are met – be they psychological or social – they are more likely to be satisfied with their working environment.

We know that lower rates of job satisfaction are associated with mental and physical ill health, higher levels of perceived stress and taking sick leave. Low job satisfaction can affect performance.

One study of job satisfaction in nurses found that practice nurses were 'highly' satisfied with their jobs and that district nurses were 'reasonably' satisfied.[3] Health visitors were 'considerably less' satisfied. The reasons given for health visitors' dissatisfaction were as follows: their work not being appreciated or valued; the fact that health promotion does not have immediate feedback as it is a long-term investment; being misunderstood by management; lack of management support; and their role being generally poorly understood. Many of the community nurses saw management as having priorities which conflicted with their own. The study indicated that nurses' job satisfaction might be eroded as they spent a greater proportion of their time on paperwork, administration and bureaucracy.

Job satisfaction can be promoted through continuing professional education and development, and opportunities for career advancement.

EXERCISE 1   Reflect back on why you chose your particular career as a nurse.

Think back and remember how and why you came to choose to be a nurse rather than opting for a different career. Did you make a positive choice or did you just drift into it? Write down all the positive reasons you had for making your career choice when you were younger. Mark against them whether they still apply or whether circumstances have changed. Have you lost sight of the positive side of the work that attracted you in the first place?

Reasons for choosing nursing   *Do they still apply?*

-

-

-

-

-

The spectrum of support and development for pursuing professional and job satisfaction

Continuing personal and professional development are integral to maintaining job satisfaction and professional fulfilment. The table below illustrates the possibilities for underpinning an individual's well-being with education and support activities, and describes the broad picture of measures that can be adopted to enhance well-being and fulfilment as a nurse.

Serious health problems	Moderate/mild depression, anxiety or stress	Well-being and personal or professional development	Professional or career fulfilment
See your GP (make time for it)	Support systems	Stress management	Career development
Referral to a specialist	Counselling	Social networking	Well-planned career path
Rehabilitation	See your GP	Team-building	Good job fit
		Communication	Rewards for performance
		Assertiveness	Learning new skills
		Time management	Clinical supervision
		Continuing education	

EXERCISE 2   Do you spend sufficient time on education and support activities?

Hopefully you are either consciously or unconsciously competent at work as far as is possible. The problem is that the focus on evidence-based practice has made people realise how little we do with regard to work for which there is hard evidence, so that we may be unconsciously incompetent at work more often than we realise. Nurses who are over-stressed may slip into conscious incompetence as they cut corners or ignore patients' emotional cues as a poor way of coping with patients' demands.

Are you satisfied with how you learn? Do you know what your preferred learning style is? Some people who prefer project work do best compiling a portfolio of new material, while others prefer to read quietly by themselves, and some prefer to attend lectures, not all of which are inspirational. If you are aware of your learning style, you can choose the educational events that suit you best.

Write down what activities you have actively sought or undertaken in the last month, that come under the umbrella of the type of activities described in the columns 'Well-being and personal or professional development' or 'Professional or career fulfilment' in the table above:

-
-
-
-

How much time have you spent on these education or support activities?

Do you think you have invested sufficient time during the last month in developing your job and skills?

Could you make more time for professional development? How and when will you start?

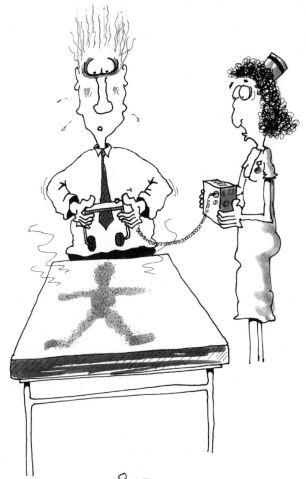

LEARN AND TRAIN PROPERLY BEFORE
PRACTISING NEW SKILLS!

▼

Practice makes perfect.

EXERCISE 3   Find out what your sources of job satisfaction are and how you compare with other people.

This exercise is divided into two parts and so, before starting the exercise, please make five photocopies of the unused table below and continued overleaf.

The first part of the exercise involves you completing the exercise for yourself. For the second part you are being asked to conduct the same exercise with five other colleagues, preferably of different grades. However, if you are unable to get different grades of nurses, this does not matter so long as you manage to involve five other colleagues. You may be wondering 'why five, and what is so magical about that number?' There is nothing magical about it other than that it will give you a reasonable number with which you can compare your personal results. Of course, the more colleagues you involve, the more likely you are to get a representative picture. One benefit of this exercise is that it will allow you to talk about job satisfaction with others, and, in addition to exchanging ideas, the exercise itself may help to relieve stress by creating opportunities for discussion.

Please note that the factors identified in the table are not listed in any order of priority. Simply indicate which of the items listed give *you* most satisfaction at work.

Please score each factor according to how important a source of satisfaction you think it is for you, from 'no satisfaction' to 'moderately satisfying' or 'very satisfying'. Please add alternative sources of satisfaction for you, that do not appear in the prepared list, to the bottom of the table.

Then repeat the exercise on five other colleagues by asking them to complete the same procedure. Compare their results with yours. The differences between you should fuel your discussions.

Source of job satisfaction	How satisfying is your job?		
	Not satisfying	Moderately satisfying	Very satisfying
Relationships with patients			
Ability to deal with patients' or clients' problems			
Relationship with staff other than nurses			
Relationship with other nurses			

EXERCISE 3   Continued.

Source of job satisfaction	How satisfying is your job?		
	Not satisfying	Moderately satisfying	Very satisfying
Job security			
Public's view of nurses			
Pay			
Continuing education – keeping up to date			
Own working conditions			
Ability to prevent illness by health promotion			
Other:			
Other:			

How did you compare with your colleagues?

What sources of job satisfaction were common to you and your colleagues (moderately or very satisfying)?

1

2

3

4

EXERCISE 4 What sources of job satisfaction could you enhance for yourself? (Give at least two)

1

2

3

4

What action do you propose to take to boost the sources of satisfaction you have just identified above, and when?

Action proposed	*Start date*
1	
2	
3	
4	

MOTIVATION

People are motivated by different things, and arguments rage as to whether anyone is ever driven by entirely altruistic motives. The following are the best motivators for fulfilling people's needs:

- interesting and/or useful work

- a sense of achievement

- responsibility

- the opportunity for career progression or professional development

- gaining new skills and competencies

- a sense of belonging (to a professional group, employing organisation or workplace team).

A study of young people's work ethic has found that 'Generation X' (the 18 to 29 year age group) wants stimulating work, variety, to be learning constantly and to receive continuous feedback on how they are doing.[6] Other studies of job satisfaction in organisations in general show that employees rate achievement, recognition, responsibility, advancement and growth more highly than salary, status, security, supervision, relationships with work colleagues and work conditions.

Pride, lust, anger, gluttony, envy, sloth and covetousness are all listed as prime motivators – hopefully not all of these are relevant to any great extent in nursing. Money motivates many people, but job satisfaction and being valued matter more to some people than money alone. As someone once said, 'money may get you to work, but it does not guarantee that you will do the job well once you are there'.

Maslow's hierarchy of human needs describes how self-esteem and fulfilment are not possible if the basic structure and safety components of your life are not secure.[7] Self-esteem encompasses self-respect, status and recognition from others. The latter three components are only possible if they are built on a good social base that includes love, friendship, belonging to groups (work, home, leisure, professional), and social activities. Fulfilment, maturity and wisdom are only possible in a person when all of the other conditions in their life encourage growth, personal development and accomplishment. Your managers in general have a responsibility to create a working environment in which motivation can occur and needs can be met.

EXERCISE 5 What mainly motivates you?

Once you have achieved an income in your family unit that gives you a reasonable standard of living, what would you say that you are mainly motivated by? (e.g. money, helping people) Write down the top three motivators as applied to your job:

-

-

-

GETTING THE RIGHT BALANCE IN YOUR JOB

The following exercises describe features of work that nurses frequently identify as important aspects of their work and job satisfaction. Make an assessment of how satisfied you are with your current job by completing the exercises below, reviewing the implications of your responses, and making a plan if you can see that there is a need to make changes.

EXERCISE 6 Review how satisfied you are with the amount of money you earn (taking into account income from others with whom you live).

- Do you earn an appropriate amount for your or your family unit's needs?

(*Too much/Appropriate/Too little*)

Review: If you feel that you earn too much or too little, do you want to plan to increase or decrease your income?

So what is your plan?

- Are you content with the balance between the level of your income and free time?

(*Yes/No*)

Review: Would you be prepared to reduce your income substantially for a corresponding gain in free time or slower work pace, or do you wish to increase your income with a corresponding reduction in your free time?

So what is your plan?

Enhancing job satisfaction

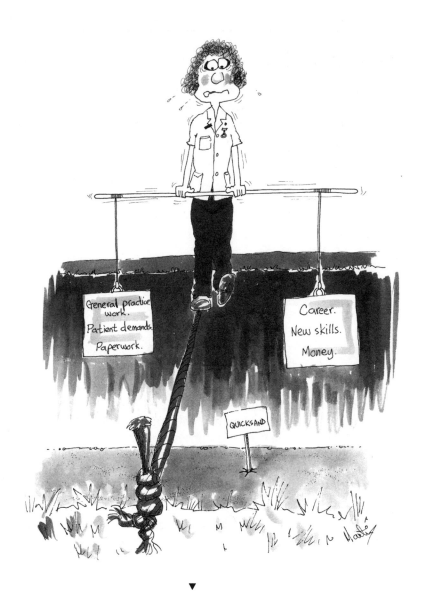

Get the right balance in your job.

EXERCISE 7   Look at opportunities for personal and professional development (at work).

- Do you have sufficient opportunities to learn new skills, undertake education, and network with other like-minded nursing colleagues? (*Yes/No*)

Review: If you do not have sufficient opportunities for professional development, what do you need to do? (create dedicated time, identify contacts or experts, find resources such as course fees, find sources of information describing the range of opportunities and how to progress?)

So what is your plan?

- How motivated are you as a nurse about pursuing professional development consistently?

(*Well motivated/Indifferent/Hostile to the idea of continuing professional development*)

Review: If you are indifferent or hostile to continuing professional development, is this because you are stressed or burnt out, or do you feel that your performance cannot be bettered and there is nothing you don't know, or do you just never get round to prioritising time for professional development? Is there any way or any person with whom you can explore the underlying reasons for your not embracing a professional development culture? What about visiting a stress counsellor, or your professional body for career guidance, e.g. the National Boards for Nursing, Midwifery and Health Visiting, or someone in education or a time-management specialist?

So what is your plan?

EXERCISE 8   To what extent do you use your skills, knowledge and experience?

- How often do you use the majority of your skills, knowledge and experience as a nurse or health professional? (*Every day/Most days/Once a week/Occasionally*)

Review: In what ways might you utilise your skills, knowledge and experience better in your current workplace? Will it require substantial changes to make more use of your skills, knowledge and experience without moving outside your workplace? Would it be worth the effort of expanding your horizons and doing at least something outside your workplace in order to make more use of your skills, knowledge and experience?

So what is your plan?

EXERCISE 9   How contented are you with the interpersonal relationships at work?

- Do you like your colleagues at work, and do they like you?

(*Yes, usually/Indifferent/Actively dislike*)

- To what extent do you need to feel liked by everybody?
  (*Yes, usually/Indifferent*)

Review: Does constantly aiming to be liked interfere with your feeling comfortable at work, and does it force you to behave unnaturally? If work colleagues dislike each other, is there anything you can do to build a team spirit through group activities at work or social events outside work?

So what is your plan?

- To what extent do you respect your work colleagues and do they respect you? (*Usually respect each other/One-sided respect/Mutually disrespectful*)

Review: Are you content with the situation? Is there anything else you might do to build up your colleagues' respect for you, or at least to cease losing their respect?

So what is your plan?

EXERCISE 10   How reasonable is your workload?

- How does the level of demands that make up your workload seem to you?

(*Too much/About right/Too little*)

- Is there a good balance between the proportion that is routine and that which is stimulating or challenging? (*Good balance/Poor balance*)

- Is the workload distributed well throughout your working day?

(*Usually well distributed/Mixed or unpredictable*)

Review: What else might be done to maintain your workload at reasonably consistent levels? How many of these alterations are within your control?

So what is your plan?

EXERCISE 11   How satisfied are you with your working hours?

- How satisfied are you with your working hours, including the number of hours and timing?

(*Usually contented/Indifferent/Usually discontented*)

Review: If you are discontented or think your working hours could be improved, what else might be done to achieve better working hours? How many of these changes are within your control?

So what is your plan?

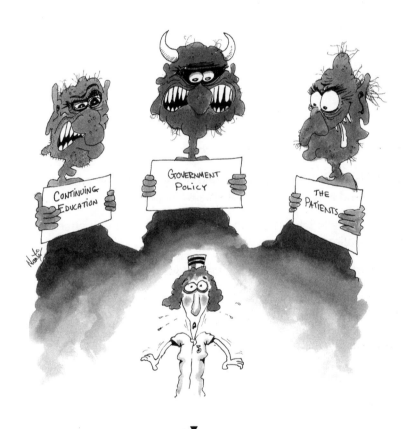

▼

Controlling your work.

EXERCISE 12   How satisfied are you with the degree of participation or control you have over your work?

- How satisfied are you with the extent to which you are involved in decision-making at work? (*Generally satisfied/Seldom satisfied/Not satisfied*)

Review: If you are dissatisfied, what else could you do to improve your involvement in decision-making at any or all levels of your organisation?

So what is your plan?

- Does your organisation have a mission statement, set of values or a development plan? If so, do you know what they are?

Review: Are you as aware as you might be of what the intended direction of your organisation is?

So what is your plan?

EXERCISE 13   How satisfied are you with the amount of time you spend in contact with patients or clients?

- How satisfied are you with the amount of time you spend in contact with patients?

(*Generally satisfied/Seldom satisfied/Not satisfied*)

Review: If you are dissatisfied, what else can you do to increase contact with patients or clients?

So what is your plan?

EXERCISE 14   To what extent are you satisfied with the level of your core skills?

- What are your communication skills like? Have you become more complacent about how you talk to patients, their relatives or student nurses? Can you switch into different styles intentionally to suit the three groups of people and their circumstances, or are you stuck in a communication rut?

(*Good communicator/Fair communicator/Poor communicator*)

- What about new skills, such as your level of computer literacy? Do you have basic keyboard skills, i.e. do you type with more than two fingers? (*Yes/Some/No*)

Review: There are many skills and competencies which, once gained, make your job easier and give you a sense of pride and achievement. Make a mental list now of what core skills you have, and which you should try to learn. Here is an opportunity to resolve to learn those skills you have been meaning to get round to some day.

So what is your plan?

EXERCISE 15   How satisfied are you with the organisation of your work setting?

- Does everything run smoothly? How satisfied are you with the way in which your workplace is organised? (*Very satisfied/Moderately satisfied/Not at all satisfied*)

- Is your workplace well managed, with good practices such as induction for new staff, regular job appraisals for all staff, attention to healthy working, and adequate staff training?

(*Well managed/Fairly well managed/Not at all well managed*)

Review: For a well-organised person, there is nothing more frustrating than trying to work amidst chaos if few people know where things are kept, forms are found in several places, the handover report either takes too long or never starts on time, patients' progress is not always entered in the nursing notes, or staff forget to pass on messages or turn up late for work. A well-managed workplace gives people clarity of purpose in their roles.

So what is your plan?

IMPROVING SATISFACTION WITH YOUR ENVIRONMENT

Working in a disturbing or unpleasant physical environment is likely to cause you stress and, conversely, working in a restful pleasing environment will reduce stress.

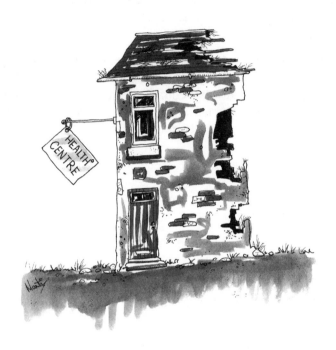

▼
Your environment.

EXERCISE 16   Reviewing your workplace.

Go round your current workplace and check it out.

- Make a list of the things that would increase the comfort of everyone working there. For example, are there enough chairs available for people to sit on?

- Is there somewhere easily accessible for private conversation about patients or clients or colleagues?

- Is the lighting adequate when it is dark outside? Do you need extra lighting for carrying out clinical procedures?

- Do smells from dirty feet, bad breath or unwashed bodies hang around? Can you improve the air flow or import a better background smell?

- Are the windows thick enough to exclude external noise sufficiently? Could you muffle noise more by arranging different ventilation or requesting secondary double-glazing?

- Does the place need freshening up, a different colour scheme or pictures on the wall?

- Is there anything you can glance up at when the going gets tough and you want to cheer yourself up – pithy sayings, funny cartoons, witty books?

So what is your plan? What changes will you make to your environment?

DEVELOPING A POSITIVE ATTITUDE TO YOUR WORKING LIFE

Job satisfaction is very much to do with your attitude to work and your expectations. There may be many aspects of your work that you would eliminate or change if you had a free choice. Working with a group of other colleagues will mean making compromises so that you can work together as a team. Of course, your capacity to accommodate your personal preferences will depend on the size of the team and the power structure. When you cannot have things exactly the way you want them at work, you can either be overly frustrated and chafe over the limitations, or you can develop the kind of attitude that makes the best of things with a generally positive outlook on life. Many nurses and other health-care colleagues are suffering from 'change fatigue' after the succession of recent major reorganisations within the health service. A positive outlook combats many of the frustrations resulting from so much change.

For a positive approach:

- concentrate on what you can do and not on what you cannot do
- accept your limitations – you are not superwoman or superman/ super-spouse, nor do you need to be super-houseproud
- get things in perspective – don't get overwhelmed by demands; put problems and unhappy experiences behind you
- don't feel guilty about circumstances outside your control
- smile and actively think positive thoughts
- look for the humour in a situation whenever appropriate
- seek out and encourage other positive people; avoid people who continually find fault
- value yourself for being assertive
- take pride in your achievements
- think future commitments through and visualise yourself as positively in control
- make positive plans to learn from mistakes
- communicate confidently
- use positive body language.

EXERCISE 17   Identify some positive features of your working and home lives.

Write down three examples from work which illustrate your positive outlook on life (e.g. a recent achievement):

-

-

-

Write down three examples from outside work which illustrate your positive outlook on life (e.g. pride in a skill such as sailing):

-

-

-

Is there anything you might do to think or behave in a more positive manner more often (e.g. smile more)?

-

-

-

ESTABLISHING A NETWORK OF RELATIONSHIPS WITH OTHER COLLEAGUES

Your experience will tell you that as well as being a complex organisation, the health service is also a major employer of nearly a million staff. When we talk about establishing effective working relationships with other colleagues, we are talking about those within our immediate zone of influence. Think of the clinical area or setting in which you work. Most people tend to work within teams of 8 to 12 people. Face-to-face contact with members will vary according to working patterns, and is likely to be high among those whose working hours are from 9 am to 5 pm. However, as most hospital nurses tend to work shifts and nights, they may go for weeks without seeing particular colleagues. 'Networking' may seem to be just another cliché, but it can be a powerful way of gaining support from others to achieve common goals – that is, providing better services or care for patients.

On the other hand, attending courses, conferences and study days provides valuable opportunities for getting to know other colleagues in the same field. Once contact is established, it becomes a lot easier to share thoughts and ideas with one another. One of the most common findings is that other colleagues are experiencing similar problems or issues. The feeling of not being alone can be very reassuring in that it helps to dispel the myth that everybody else has got it right except you. It can also encourage individuals to take positive action to address their dissatisfaction by hearing how others have done so. Good partnerships with colleagues don't just happen unless you are very lucky – they usually have to be worked at. In a small working environment, colleagues can stop supporting each other for many reasons, but often it is because of unwillingness to give and take. For example, the manager who wants staff to be flexible with their shifts will not get very far if there is no gain for the staff.

Job satisfaction is very much an individual matter. Although most people will put happiness above money, when it comes to work, money remains a powerful factor. However, it is the non-monetary factors that most people tend to cite when they talk about being dissatisfied at work. These factors range from not being valued to inflexibility and unrealistic expectations and demands. In the end it is important that we exercise the choice we all have – to seek a job that will meet the needs we cherish most. Of course, changing career is one option. Module 6 covers ideas for career development or even a career change. If you really are irreversibly dissatisfied with your current job, why not work through the next Module soon?

EXERCISE 18   Compare your circumstances and workplace with others where nursing staff say they are satisfied with the job they do.

Talk to your colleagues and list the features which they think contribute to their job satisfaction:

-

-

-

-

How many of those features exist within your workplace?

Which of the sources of job satisfaction that are present for other nurses, but not for you, can you import to your workplace or your own situation?

References

1 Wade B (1993) The job satisfaction of health visitors, district nurses and practice nurses working in areas served by four trusts: year 1. *J Adv Nurs*. **18**: 992–1004.

2 Ootim B (1998) Self-esteem. *Nurs Manage*. **4**: 24–5.

3 Muncey T (1998) Selection and retention of nurses. *J Adv Nurs*. **27**: 406–13.

4 Hinde J (1998) Nurses are not carrying on. *The Times Higher Educational Supplement*, 27 November.

5 Fung-Kam L (1998) Job satisfaction and autonomy of Hong Kong registered nurses. *J Adv Nurs*. **27**: 355–63.

6 Cannon D (1996) *Generation X and the new work ethic*. Demos, London.

7 Maslow AH (1970) *Motivation and personality*. Harper and Row, New York.

Further reading

Bailey R (1998) Attendance allowance. *Occup Health.* **50**: 23–5.

Castledine G (1998) How to improve the morale of nursing students. *Br J Nurs.* **7**: 290.

Garbett R (1998) It's tough at the top. *Nurs Times.* **94**: 68–9.

Girvin J (1998) Satisfaction and motivation. *Nurs Manage.* **5**: 11–15.

Hancock C (1998) Keeping staff means demonstrating to nurses that they matter. *Nurs Times Res.* **3**: 165–6.

Landy C (1998) Valuing your staff. *Nurs Manage.* **5**: 20–1.

Mangan P (1998) One in four nurse directors feels undervalued. *Br J Nurs.* **7**: 754.

Mashta O (1998) Time to go. *Nurs Standard.* **12**: 12–13.

Nolan M, Brown J, Naughton M *et al.* (1998) Developing nursing future. Role 2. Nurses' job satisfaction and morale. *Br J Nurs.* **7**: 1044–8.

Parry-Jones B, Grant G, McGrath M *et al.* (1998) Stress and job satisfaction among social workers, community nurses and community psychiatric nurses: implications for the care management model. *Health Soc Care Commun.* **6**: 271–85.

Robinson S, Murrells T (1998) Getting started: choice and constraint in obtaining a post after qualifying as a registered mental nurse. *J Nurs Manage.* **6**: 137–46.

Stephen H (1998) How much are you worth? *Nurs Standard.* **13**: 14–15.

MODULE 6
Promoting career development

AIMS

The aims of Module 6 are:

1 To improve awareness of nursing career options.

2 To increase nurses' understanding of the opportunities for career development.

3 To engage nurses in reflecting on their own career development to date.

4 To encourage nurses actively to plan the rest of their careers.

CONTENTS

Starting to think about career development
- Career planning.
  Exercise 1: Think back to reflect on how much of a role chance has played in your career path (time to be taken = 15 mins).
- Understand your own career preferences and style.
  Exercise 2: How well matched are you to your current nursing job? (time to be taken = 30 mins).
  Exercise 3: Review your current job, qualifications and interests (time to be taken = 1 hour).

Professional development opportunities
- ENB key characteristics.
  Exercise 4: To what extent have you met the ENB's key characteristics? (time to be taken = 1 hour).
- Specialist nursing practice.
- Being involved in the training and education of nurses.
- Working as a nurse practitioner.
- Working as a clinical nurse specialist.
- Portfolio nursing careers.

Flexible working
  Exercise 5: Decide whether increasing the flexibility of your current post might suit you (time to be taken = 10 mins).
- Types of flexible working.
- Disadvantages of flexible working.

Other career options
  Exercise 6: Which of the alternative nursing career areas described above appeal to you? (time to be taken = 15 mins).
- The advantages and disadvantages of taking on a job outside your workplace.

Gaining nursing careers information, advice, guidance or counselling
  Exercise 7: Do you know where you could obtain careers information, advice, guidance or counselling? (time to be taken = 20 mins).
- Find a buddy, mentor or coach.
  Exercise 8: With whom could you discuss your career development? (time to be taken = 20 mins).

And finally

Exercise 9: Reassess your current job (time to be taken = 1 hour).

The total time needed to work through this module will depend on the amount of time you spend reflecting on how the information in the module applies to you, before completing the exercises. The total time that it might take to complete this module is 6 hours (including time for reading, reflecting, and completing the exercises).

Below are the comments made by some participants at a career development course about their experiences.

'The course had a great impact on me. A significant part of my life previously was my career ... the course has given me confidence in my personal abilities and my thinking and my decision-making.'

'I am considering other career options in research and teaching'.

'The course ... broadened horizons within nursing, made me more keen.'

'Raised my awareness of the wide range of opportunities possible within nursing.'

'Made me aware of what I could be doing.'

'People set themselves up for failure and sabotage themselves in a million different ways.'

'Opened up my eyes to other opportunities I hadn't thought of before.'

'Gave me a jolt to realise in how limited a way I'd been thinking.'

'Set me on the route to success.'

STARTING TO THINK ABOUT CAREER DEVELOPMENT

You wouldn't be reading this book unless you were wondering if there is anything you can do to enhance or change your career. You may just be seeking reassurance that you are reasonably content in your current job, or alternatively you may want to review your whole career, feeling that working in your present nursing role is not for you. You may just want to check out what other opportunities exist. You may be finding that the other pressures in your life are just too much in combination with a busy nursing life, whether they involve looking after young children or elderly dependents, or struggling to cope with your own physical or mental ill health, or other unsettling personal events.

This module should appeal to any nurse who wants a career check-up. It should be useful for those nurses who wonder if the grass is greener elsewhere or want to expand their horizons, for those contemplating a career in other settings, such as a return to acute settings, or moving to nursing posts in community or primary care settings, or for nurses wondering about other options within nursing, such as nurse education, management, research or developing a specialism. This book should also appeal to those in nursing who advise others about their career options, and those nurses who have personal reasons for wanting to develop their career while looking after young children or coping with ill health. The majority of nurses working in the NHS have caring responsibilities,[1] with 41% having dependent children, 16% having dependent adults and 4% having both.

Fulfilment and personal growth top Maslow's hierarchy of needs,[2] and are only likely to occur if the basics of an individual's life are in place – security, social networks, etc. If you are contemplating a career change or expansion of your career that will require new skills, knowledge and experience, you might be better off waiting until your personal life is reasonably settled and you feel secure before making major alterations or moving on.

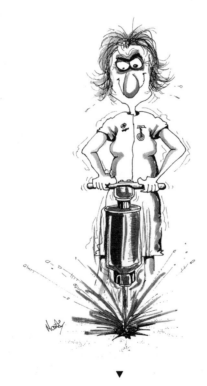

▼

Preparing the ground to make the most of your career.

The lack of a clear career structure is a well-recognised cause of stress in any workforce, not just nursing, although the current climate of change and uncertainty also contributes to stress in nurses.[3] The majority of nursing students entering adult and children's branches of preregistration nurse training are under 26 years old.[4] These entrants may be more idealistic about what nursing involves, have comparatively less life experience, and be unaware of the range of career opportunities within nursing. Similarly, some nurses reach their top grade within several years of entering practice, to find a flat career structure and no obvious route to promotion. NHS managers may think that they have a career structure, only to find that the NHS reorganisation changes such that there is no obvious career progression and they need to transfer to a different pathway in another setting.

An additional stress for some nurses is that they may not be working in their preferred specialism or setting. Some nurses leave the care setting they prefer because they find that their unsocial hours and working shifts are incompatible with other caring responsibilities, such as raising a family or looking after an elderly relative. Other nurses may find the opposite is true, that they are trapped in their current post because the working patterns allow them to work around their domestic responsibilities. If you are not working in your chosen nursing career specialty, you may be less likely to find your job satisfying and more likely to be stressed.

The Royal College of Nursing (RCN) is concerned about the shortfall in applications for nurse education places. In 1996–1997 there were 15 400 applications for 16 100 places at university departments. The number of new nurses registering to practise has declined year on year for a decade. About one-third of nursing students drop out during the preregistration course. The RCN is calling for twice as many nurses to be trained in order to meet the expected need and current vacancies. In addition, the Department of Health wants to boost the numbers of nurses on diploma and degree courses by 6000 in the next 3 years in the 49 universities in the UK that offer such courses. More than half of those on the nursing register are aged 40 years or over.

Men constitute about 11% of nursing students,[5] and just over 9% of nurses registered with the UKCC. It has been reported that 88 of 32 800 practising midwives are male.[5]

In total, 4300 of the 6000 applications from outside the European Union for registration as a nurse were successful in the 12-month period up to 31 March 1998.[5]

Career planning

The key to career planning is information-gathering from people, books and general observation. By conducting your career by chance rather than by thoughtful planning you end up taking opportunities as they come along, rather than taking control and finding the best match of career to your own needs and preferences.

It is difficult to plan your career and make informed choices about which nursing specialty you will opt for if you have not taken advantage of the nursing career counselling services that are available to nursing students and qualified nurses, or if your experience of alternative nursing specialties is limited.

Career planning is about career growth, and the pathway along which you learn more about yourself, the facts about the options open to you, the implications of the alternative posts in terms of training, career progression, workload, etc., how to gain qualifications or equip yourself educationally for your preferred posts, how to manage the transition period while taking up new posts, and subsequently how to review and develop your career.

There is a wide range of career options available to nurses today

If you wish to switch careers or combine a substantial new post with your current nursing post, you should plan ahead and go for a gradual transition rather than an impulsive change. Your previous experience should have paved the way for you to have a good understanding of the types of work and ways of working that suit you. The more the different components of your nursing career overlap and you can carry your various skills and strengths over to your chosen post, the easier it is to break new ground from your relatively confident position.

All nurses need career planning at every stage of their careers. Many nurses still enjoy the job they do and the post they hold, but those responsible for planning workforce developments should consider the potential for retaining nurses in innovative ways with secondments and new nursing developments (e.g. nurse practitioners working with homeless people). Although nurses can retire at 55 years of age, this is often the time when they have built up a wealth of expertise and skills. This you can demonstrate through your professional portfolio. You may have less energy as you get older, but your additional experience should make up for that, so there is no reason why someone in their fifties cannot perform as well as if not better than a young nurse. You will have fewer financial and domestic pressures as the family grow up and leave home, and you will be able to focus more on your work (if you want to!)

EXERCISE 1   Think back to reflect on how much of a role chance has played in your own career path.

To what extent is it due to chance or an unexpected opportunity that you trained for nursing, or that you work in the setting you do? Write down your reflections on how much was due to chance, and whether there is any other job you might like to be doing now if you had planned your career differently:

On balance, are you happy with your current career choice? (*Yes/No*)

If no, is it too late to change career track now, or could you combine your current job with another career activity related to the other choice of career? What do you think? (Be realistic!)

Understanding your own career preferences and style

You cannot make a rational career choice without understanding the 'inner you' and what you have to offer. Your career and personality match are very important – and your personal preferences for the balance between work and leisure, work and income, degree of responsibility, type of work, and extent of interaction with people.

There are many varieties of personality profile questionnaires. Two of the best known are the Myers-Briggs type indicator,[6] which measures four bipolar dimensions of personality, and the 16PF questionnaire, which assesses 16 personality factors. In one *Return to Work* course, most of the participants rated the workshop session where they received feedback on their Myers-Briggs scores as one of the best of the year's course. For many of them, becoming more aware of their personal preferences and styles meant that they gained confidence and pride in their own characteristics, rather than seeking to conform to a nursing stereotype. Many thought that understanding themselves better would help them to find posts where they were more likely to fit comfortably into the setting and requirements of the job.

Although nursing offers a wide spectrum of opportunities which extend beyond the traditional posts, many nurses who develop too far away from their core specialty eventually feel disconnected without their 'career anchor', and want some direct contact with nursing practice.[7] They find that they need to keep in touch and literally 'keep their hand in'. There are plenty of ex-nurses who have moved on to such diverse jobs as nursing advisers to health authorities, newspaper journalists, or civil servants who continue to do regular nursing shifts not just to maintain their credibility with their peers or to keep themselves up to date or their options open for return, but also to stay connected with the core career anchor in their lives.

Eight career anchor categories have been identified by Schein and used to increase people's insights about their strengths and motivation in career development, namely technical or functional competence, general managerial competence, autonomy or independence, security or stability, entrepreneurial creativity, service or dedication to a cause, pure challenge and lifestyle.[7] People define their self-image in terms of these traits, and come to understand more about their talents, motives and values – and which of these is so important to them that they would not give up those facets of themselves if forced to make a choice.

EXERCISE 2   How well matched are you to your current nursing job?

How well does your personality suit your current job?
(*Very well/Moderately/Not at all well*)

What three key attributes about you personally match the requirements of your job (go on – sing your own praises, don't be humble):

-

-

-

What do you particularly like about the nature of your job? (e.g. being with people, helping people, etc.)

What is your 'career anchor' – that is, of the list described by Schein above, what is the one feature about you and your job that you would not give up, no matter what?

- technical or functional competence

- general managerial competence

- autonomy or independence

- security or stability

- entrepreneurial creativity

- service or dedication to a cause

- pure challenge

- lifestyle.

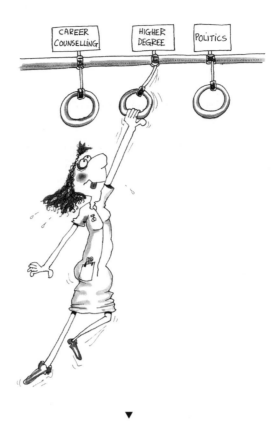

▼
Career change.

EXERCISE 3   Reviewing your current job, qualifications and interests can help you to identify your future professional development needs and priorities.

Work through your professional portfolio, making sure that it is up to date.

While doing this you may find that a theme for the focus of your nursing work emerges. Your own personal interest in some aspects of your role as a nurse often reveals areas which you want to develop further. Your theme may be counselling, health promotion or working with a particular client group.

Write in your portfolio the themes which emerge for you. You may have more than one theme.

PROFESSIONAL DEVELOPMENT OPPORTUNITIES

Education and training opportunities

There is a wide range of options available for nurses in the UK. There are three main categories of courses, namely clinical, academic and professional courses. Most courses are offered by Schools of Nursing in universities, and are modular and credit rated. A module is a discrete unit of study which may be offered as a free-standing unit or as part of a course. Credits are awarded when students successfully complete a module, and these credits can be combined to create a specific academic award such as a diploma or a degree. Credits can be at Level One, corresponding to the first year of a degree, Level Two, corresponding to the second year of a degree, or Level Three, corresponding to the third year of an honours degree. The fourth level of credits, sometimes referred to as Level M, corresponds to Masters level studies. Although credits can be added together to form a diploma or a degree, there are certain criteria which are specific to each university, so it is important that you obtain advice about combining modules for this purpose before you have accumulated 60 credits. Contact your local School of Nursing for more information about these opportunities.

The type of professional development which is appropriate to you is dependent on a number of factors which are individual to each nurse. These include your previous training and experience, your academic qualifications, the level and type of clinical responsibility you have, and the development plans of your employing organisation.

You will need to discuss the kinds of courses and training you want to pursue with your employer, colleagues, mentor/buddy or your National Board. Funding is more likely if the course you want to pursue will meet some of the needs of your employing organisation.

The English National Board (ENB) provides a wide range of careers advice, both in booklet form and via its web page. It has extensive information relating to post-registration career development, and the Board is able to provide enquirers with information about health-related graduate and postgraduate courses from the ECCTIS 2000 computer database.

The ENB has accredited over 169 different courses, different combinations of which are offered by various Schools of Nursing in different universities. For further information, surf the ENB web page which contains information relating to each of the different courses, or write to your National Board specifying which courses you are interested in. Similar services are also offered by the Welsh, Scottish and Northern Ireland National Boards.

The ENB Framework For Continuing Professional Education, and its Higher Award for Nurses, Midwives and Health Visitors,[8] aim to provide a flexible and coherent system for continuing professional education to enable nurses to work towards the ENB Higher Award, which is both a professional and an academic qualification. This opportunity has been developed to enable nurses working in both acute and community settings to demonstrate real expertise in clinical skills and professional knowledge.

This ENB Framework provides a foundation for the implementation of the United Kingdom Central Council's Standards for Education and Practice following initial nurse registration.[8] The framework builds upon 10 key characteristics which are listed below.[8]

ENB key characteristics[8]

1 Professional accountability and responsibility

2 Clinical expertise with a specific client group

3 Use of research to plan, implement and evaluate strategies to improve care

4 Team working and building and multidisciplinary team leadership

5 Flexible and innovative approaches to care

6 Use of health-promotion strategies

7 Facilitating and assessing development in others

8 Handling information and making informed clinical decisions

9 Setting standards and evaluating quality of care

10 Initiating, managing and evaluating clinical change.

These 10 key characteristics provide a benchmark against which all nurses can examine their practice and plan an individual programme of professional development. The ENB does offer a professional portfolio which you can use to plan your overall professional development. If you want to gain the formal qualification of ENB Higher Award, you can do so using the 10 key characteristics as the basis. However, you will also need to register with a Board-approved School of Nursing and to index with the Board. In addition, you will need to negotiate learning contracts with your manager and educationalists and have the help of a practice supervisor.

EXERCISE 4   To what extent have you fulfilled the ENB's key characteristics?

Take each of the characteristics in turn and identify any examples from your practice which you consider show that you have that characteristic. You may have trouble identifying any examples initially. However, if you think about your practice and perhaps discuss this with your mentor or buddy, you may see that some or all of the characteristics are a feature of your work or experience.

	ENB key characteristics[8]	My examples from practice
1	Professional accountability and responsibility	
2	Clinical expertise with a specific client group	
3	Use of research to plan, implement and evaluate strategies to improve care	
4	Team working and building and multidisciplinary team leadership	
5	Flexible and innovative approaches to care	
6	Use of health-promotion strategies	
7	Facilitating and assessing development in others	
8	Handling information and making informed clinical decisions	
9	Setting standards and evaluating quality of care	
10	Initiating, managing and evaluating clinical change	

Specialist nursing practice

Knowing what you want to be doing in 5 years' time enables you to identify professional development opportunities. There is a wide range of options available to you as a nurse.

The United Kingdom Central Council (UKCC) for Nursing, Midwifery and Health Visiting states that preregistration nursing education equips newly qualified nurses to provide safe and effective care in hospitals and other institutions in the community.[9] Usually this is as a staff nurse.

The UKCC has defined the characteristics of specialist nursing practice.[9] At this level of professional practice, higher levels of expertise are expected in clinical decision-making skills, and the monitoring and improvement of standards of care through the supervision of practice, clinical audit, developing and leading practice, contributing to research and teaching and supporting other professional colleagues are demonstrated. Specialist practitioners work in a variety of community and acute-care settings. In 1994, the UKCC identified eight specialist areas of practice for community health care nursing.[9] These were as follows:

- general practice nursing
- occupational health care nursing
- community children's nursing
- public health nursing
- school nursing
- community nursing in the home – district nursing
- community mental health nursing
- community mental handicap nursing.

Specialist areas of practice in acute-care settings are still evolving, although there have been developments in the following specialist nurse areas:

- accident and emergency
- theatres
- gerontology
- oncology
- palliative care
- renal care.

The UKCC is currently debating the criteria for nurses to demonstrate that they are working at a Higher Level of Practice.[9] This level is based on clinical competency, and is to be determined locally and related to particular areas of nursing practice. This level of practice supports the concepts of clinical governance and lifelong learning. For further clarification of higher and advanced levels of nursing practice, contact your National Board.

In addition to this pathway of professional development opportunities for nurses, there are many others, as described below.

Involvement in the training and education of nurses

Nursing education and training are rapidly changing. The UKCC has recently published standards relating to the preparation of nurses who are involved in education and training.[10] Four clearly identified roles and functions relate to this area. These are:

- mentors and mentorship
- preceptors and preceptorship
- practice educator and practice education
- lecturers and education.

These four roles are described more fully below.

Mentors and mentorship

Mentoring provides support, guidance and role models for students in the nursing workplace.

Preceptors

Preceptors are tutors who work with students and provide support in the workplace.

Practice educators and practice education

Practice educators are experienced practitioners with a broad understanding of clinical practice, who make a significant contribution to the education of students and practitioners, identify the professional development needs of the team and ensure that they are met, and lead the development of practice within their practice settings.

Lecturers and education

Lecturers should be regarded as practitioners who undertake their substantive teaching role in a higher education setting and who contribute to learning activity in practice settings.

The criteria which should be met for these roles are identified in the right-hand column of the table below.

Role	Criteria
Mentor	Effective registration with the UKCC
	12 months of full-time experience (or equivalent part-time)
	Support for role
	Access to lecturer or practice educator
	Support from line manager
Preceptor	Effective registration with the UKCC
	12 months (or equivalent part-time) of experience within the same or associated clinical fields as the practitioner requiring support
Practice Educator	Effective registration with the UKCC
	Completed minimum 3 years of full-time experience (or equivalent part-time) in relevant professional practice in the last 10 years
	Acquired additional professional knowledge relevant to area of practice at no lower than degree level
	The programme of study leading to the qualification of practice educator must be at no lower than degree level
	Community practitioners teachers' course, or an equivalent course
	Portfolio of evidence
Lecturer	Effective registration with the UKCC
	Completed minimum 3 years of full-time experience (or equivalent part-time) in relevant professional practice in the last 10 years
	Acquired additional professional knowledge relevant to area of practice, at no lower than degree level
	The programme of study leading to the qualification of lecturer will be at postgraduate level

(Note that additional professional knowledge is described in a glossary of terms published by the UKCC as follows.[10] 'It is essential that a teacher can demonstrate a level of knowledge of the subject above that which the student is required to learn. Such knowledge can be achieved in a number of ways. For example, either through a taught course or presentation of a portfolio for academic accreditation or a combination of the two.')

Working as a nurse practitioner

There is some confusion about the title of 'nurse practitioner'. A recent survey found that nurses described themselves as nurse practitioners without having undertaken specific training.[11] This is influenced in part by the fact that within the UK the role of nurse practitioner has been a recent development and has yet to be recognised by the UKCC. The title 'nurse practitioner', according to the Royal College of Nursing, describes a nurse with the extra knowledge and skills that allow her or him to practise in areas that have previously been viewed as the traditional preserve of physicians.[12] In 1996, the Royal College of Nursing agreed that preparation of nurse practitioners should be at first-degree level.[12]

The Royal College of Nursing outlines the role as one where the nurse practitioner:

* makes professionally accountable decisions for which she or he has sole responsibility.

* receives patients or clients with undifferentiated and undiagnosed problems. An assessment of their health-care needs is based on highly developed nursing knowledge and skills. This includes special skills not usually exercised by nurses, such as physical examination.

* screens for disease risk factors and early signs of illness.

* develops a nursing care plan for health with the patient, putting an emphasis on preventative measures.

* provides counselling and health education.

* has the authority to admit or discharge patients from her or his own caseload and refer them on to other health-care providers as appropriate.

The specific admissions criteria for this course vary from one institution to another. However, the general criteria are that applicants should be registered nurses who have completed study at Level Two and achieved 120 Level Two credits or the equivalent.

For further information, contact your local universities and your National Board Careers Advice service.

Clinical nurse specialist

Clinical nurse specialist roles have been in place since the 1970s, especially in areas such as infection control, tissue viability, stoma care and continence.[13] Nurses undertaking these roles have undertaken post-registration education and are recognised as experts in a particular field of care. However, the title has not been recognised by the UKCC. Nurse specialists are usually employed by NHS Trusts.

There are many post-registration educational qualifications for which the training is part-time and can theoretically be fitted in around work, although in reality this usually swallows up a lot of family time and annual leave, and requires considerable drive and commitment to succeed. Examples of the types of qualifications that can lead on to other job opportunities are given below:

* ENB 998 Teaching and assessing in clinical practice

- ENB 870 Introduction to the understanding and application of research
- Diploma in Nursing by either distance learning or day release
- BSc (Hons) Nursing
- BSc (Hons) Specialist Nursing Practice awards leading to specialist qualifications such as Community Nursing in the Home, District Nursing, Public Health Nursing – Health Visiting
- BA (Hons) Education
- Masters or Postgraduate Diploma in Nursing or Advanced Practice
- Masters in Business Affairs (MBA) or a Diploma
- Masters in Education
- Complementary medicine qualification, e.g. in acupuncture or homeopathy
- Non-nursing qualification
- Doctorate (PhD) or other research degree.

In addition to the opportunities outlined above, non-NHS care settings such as those listed below offer opportunities for clinical work:

- the blood transfusion service
- the Armed Forces
- the Prison Service
- overseas employment agencies
- charities and voluntary organisations.

Portfolio nursing careers

This is just the fashionable term for mixing and matching different posts, usually centring on health care in some way. Some people successfully run nursing and non-nursing jobs together, but usually one complements or feeds off the other. The *portfolio* description implies that the skills involved in the mix of jobs are transferable, and can be carried on afterwards to the next sequence of jobs that the individual health professional takes on.

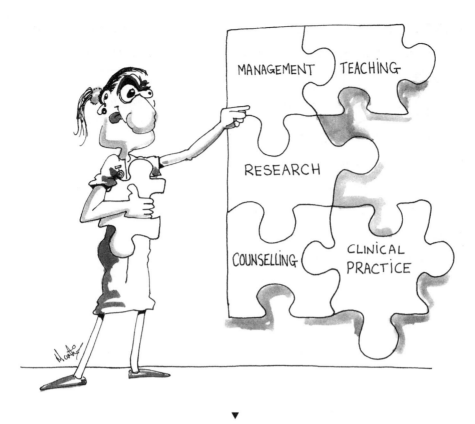

▼

Portfolio careers.

FLEXIBLE WORKING

Could you take a more flexible approach to nursing?

Flexible working may be a good way of counteracting burnout by enabling the nurse to pursue other interests and keep her or his creativity and enjoyment of nursing alive if working day after day is debilitating or a problem. Sometimes nurses earn extra money by taking on additional work outside their core job, while others are keeping their options open with a variety of jobs until they focus more specifically at some time in the future.

Flexible working is being seen as one way of solving the looming crisis in nursing workforce numbers, by increasing the attractiveness of nursing and retaining nurses who might otherwise be put off continuing working. Similarly, flexible working in medicine and other caring professions retains staff who might otherwise be unable to work due to family commitments.

Flexibility is essential if nurses are to adapt to change. Much stress in nursing arises when people resist change and blindly persist with the same traditional systems and ways of working, as if they are in a time warp. Society is constantly changing, demands and possibilities are very different now, and new ways of working are necessary if those within the profession are to survive and flourish. The UK workforce as a whole is more mobile, and more married women have a paid job than used to be the case.

Trends in UK nurses employment[1]:

- Employed in NHS nursing   70%
- Employed in non-NHS nursing   12%
- Employed by nursing agencies and banks   3%
- Taking statutory maternity leave/career breaks   3%
- Employed in GP practice   7%
- Employed in non-nursing role   1%
- Other, not defined   4%

EXERCISE 5   Decide whether increasing the flexibility of your current post might suit you.

How flexible is your working day or working week? Would you prefer that it was more flexible than it is? (*Yes/No/Don't know*)

If so, what could you do to adapt your working hours or work pattern to allow you to accommodate other work activities? (tick all that apply)

- reduce hours and seek an additional job outside your current nursing role

- change hours to liberate more blocks of time for other work (e.g. negotiate starting earlier, ending later)

- find a job-sharer

- change jobs

- find work that can be done in your spare time from home (e.g. aromatherapy, reflexology, own business).

Types of flexible working

The strengths of a portfolio career are its flexibility, variety, potential for personal development and chance to react to new opportunities or changing circumstances – either your personal circumstances or in relation to the NHS organisation. It is much better to seize the opportunities while you are on top of your job and starting to need variety and new challenges, rather than to wait until you are starting to burn out from the constant workload of being in the same nursing post long term. It is all about choice – working additional overnight shifts for a nursing home or agency involves calculating the balance between benefits and disadvantages for you as an individual and your workplace.

Flexible working patterns require flexibility from your employer as much as from the nurse concerned. The success of any innovative working arrangement depends as much on the willingness and attitudes of everyone involved as on the structure put in place as a framework to accommodate that work.

Job sharing

This normally involves two people sharing one full-time post – usually, but not necessarily, with a 50:50 split of hours, tasks and pay. Such job-sharing posts often provide a way for a full-time nursing employee to reduce her or his hours for personal or professional reasons, but sometimes a pair of nurses or other health professionals submit a joint application for an advertised vacancy and convince the interview panel that 'two heads are better than one'. Some Trusts will help nurses who are seeking potential job-share partners, and hold personal details on a database. Some job sharers divide the week in half, while others work half of each day. Sometimes job sharers cover for each other over holiday or sickness absence periods. Many have a period of overlap at least once a week to allow them to pass on messages and communicate. Some work closely as a pair, sharing the management of individual patients, while others keep their own patients or clients. There is resistance to job sharing in some Trusts, mainly by those who consider that job sharing means a lack of continuity of care, and that extra nurses confuse the patients, and who worry about filling half of a shared post if one half of the 'twosome' leaves, and the additional training costs. However, the benefits seem to outweigh the drawbacks in the majority of job-sharing arrangements, which enable nurses who are working part-time to contribute their knowledge and expertise to patient care, and to combine this with other roles and responsibilities.

Working for an agency

This option enables nurses to work flexibly, and to gain experience of a wide range of care settings while being paid to work there. This kind of working can broaden your knowledge and provide insight into a range of nursing settings. In addition to working in the NHS, agency staff also work in the independent sector, the community, nursing homes, hospices, schools and general medical practices. However, agency nurses often have limited access to study days funded by an employer, and usually have to undertake continuing education in their own time. When contracting to work for an agency, you need to ensure that you are clear about the role and responsibilities of the post you are undertaking and the rates of pay. Some agencies give holiday pay, although not all of them do so. Different Trusts and other employers will have varying rates for unsocial hours and bank-holiday working. Check the rate for the shift before doing it if you want to avoid any unpleasant surprises.

Working for a bank

Most hospital and community Trusts run their own nurse bank. A 'bank' is a database of nurses who are willing to do casual work for a Trust. One in four nurses work in this capacity in addition to their main job.[1] Quite often nurses have to ring in to register for work, although sometimes the Trust telephones them. The advantages of working for a bank are that it is local to a particular hospital or community, and continuity of care can sometimes be provided, as often 'bank' nurses work on the same ward or unit each time they are called in. Working for one employer means that these nurses can become more familiar with Trust policies and protocols. However, the disadvantages are that 'bank' nurses may be paid less for working in this way than if they worked overtime on their own ward or unit.

Disadvantages of flexible working

A major barrier to flexible working is the attitude of other nurses who scorn the part-timer or assistant for not being a 'proper' nurse. There is a lack of understanding from peers as well as from the public and patients about nurses and other health professionals who work less than full-time. Work colleagues may be suspicious of you because you are different and challenge their choice of a full-time post. Some may voice concerns that if too many nurses change to flexible working, mixing and matching various posts or specifying that they will only work between 9 am and 5 pm, there may be too few nurses left to cover the antisocial hours and do routine or behind-the-scenes work.

Many of those working in minimally part-time posts feel isolated within their workplace, especially if their working hours mean that coffee breaks and team meetings do not coincide with times when the others are free. Isolation is an issue for someone who is only one of a kind in a team, and some protected release to group education with peers can guard against such professional isolation.

Tight finances often encourage nurses to take on additional work, although this can also be a means of gaining experience in an area before committing fully to a change of post or speciality. However, casual working can mean financial insecurity, the lack of an NHS pension or sickness cover, and the drain of constantly looking for work and keeping financial records. Pay is usually relatively lower as a casual worker compared to being in a permanent post when the freelancer's lack of income while on holiday, sick or in training is taken into account.

Limited information technology (IT) skills can be a factor in making life difficult for nurses moving between paperless workplaces with varied computer systems and little induction training. This also restricts access to electronic databases of best practice, job vacancies and career advice.

Another drawback to part-time working is the lack of continuity for patients, which is rarely realised until after the change to a flexible working arrangement has been made and the nurse is spending less time in the same workplace. Nurses may feel a mixture of guilt and regret at being unavailable if patients are cared for by others when they would have previously provided 'continuity of care'.

One other aspect you should consider is what effects a new working environment may have on you, and whether these are acceptable. Nurses working at a clinical level who take on a part-time educational post seem to remain rooted in nursing practice, but those who take up management

---

positions, especially full-time positions, are often influenced by management thinking and behaviour to the extent that their nursing colleagues may feel estranged and accuse them of having lost their nursing persona. Sometimes nurses turned managers embrace their new-found management philosophy with such zeal that they outdo any dyed-in-the-wool manager for getting service costs down or other performance measures achieved.

OTHER CAREER OPTIONS

There is a wide range of posts for which nursing may be a suitable preparation and which, although not immediately obvious when considering career development, may be of interest and worth investigating further. These are described briefly in the following categories.

Advisory posts

Posts include giving expert or specialised nursing advice to health authorities, patients' organisations or the Department of Health, assisting nursing defence organisations, or working for pharmaceutical companies, computing or other commercial companies who want a nursing opinion and input, e.g. in making video films destined to be viewed by other nurses.

Information about opportunities is available from those who want the advice, or via the grapevine. Some posts are widely advertised in local and national newspapers, particularly those on public bodies that operate under the 'Nolan' rules of fair behaviour, such as non-Executive Directors of NHS Trust Boards or NHS advisory committees.

Research

Alternative ways to develop an academic career might include the following.

- Research fellows, research assistants or lecturers at Schools of Health or Departments of Nursing or Health in universities. You may be able to combine doing a job in a specific post and working for a higher degree.

- Secondments, such as a research fellowship or NHS regional training fellowships, supervised by an academic unit. You would combine your nursing job with protected time for research and undertake a higher degree attached to a supervisory academic unit. These opportunities are few and far between.

- Register for a higher degree (MPhil or PhD) with a view to gaining an academic appointment when you have obtained the research qualification.

- Join a research network that includes nurses, run by an academic unit, and participate in data collection or analysis/interpretative stages of the project, for which you may or may not be paid.

Academic success is judged by the number and quality (i.e. journal of publication) of peer-reviewed publications, the number, sources and magnitude of research grants awarded, and national recognition such as presentations at conferences, peer reviewing and membership of expert committees.

There are considerable difficulties in pursuing an academic career. These include lower pay than in many nursing-related posts, short-term contracts, opportunities not always being advertised, variable levels of departmental support, limited time for academic research and education work in nursing practice, the exorbitant costs of registration for a higher postgraduate degree, and scarcity of funds for small research projects.

Communications

These posts include writing for professional nursing journals or for the lay press, or writing books. The annual *Writers' Handbook* gives contact details for a variety of publications, indicating which of them accept unsolicited material and their pay scales. Contacting the editor and tempting them to look at your exciting outline or ideas for article(s) is usually the first step.

Speaking on the radio and television can be time-consuming and may attract little or no pay, but it can increase your profile and open the way to other work or career opportunities.

Commercial or business

In addition to the posts mentioned under the 'Advisory posts' section, you might be able to start your own company by extending a hobby or skill (e.g. computing) or a non-nursing interest (e.g. travel). Information technology and complementary medicine are both potentially good fields for starting new businesses.

Management

Another option is to combine nursing practice with management in primary care groups, with Trusts, health authorities, medical audit advisory groups, etc. There seems to be a blurred boundary between chairing and managing a body, often dependent on the extent of the infrastructure of that body and how much work can be delegated.

EXERCISE 6   Which of the alternative nursing career areas described above appeal to you?

Does any job described in this section appeal to you? (*Yes/No*)

If so, for how long have you been thinking of getting involved in that area?

What is stopping you from finding out about opportunities or taking up such a post?

Advantages and disadvantages of taking on a job outside your workplace

As well as the possible financial incentive, you will learn a lot about a different branch of nursing or from the new people you meet in the course of the other post. It is easy to get bogged down in the day-to-day stresses and demands of nursing practice, or oppressed by the more mundane aspects, and breaking out into new territory helps to keep your working life in perspective and your mind fresh. Getting outside your routine working patterns and working with other professionals who you would not normally meet gives you a broader perspective on both nursing and life in general.

You will need to make an honest assessment of why you should opt for a particular post. The effort involved in meeting the skills and responsibilities of the new post will probably be considerable, and should not be undertaken just because it happens to be available and you are flattered that someone has asked you to apply. If you foresee a good opportunity for personal development, and the potential job interests you, you might decide that the pay is of secondary importance.

GAINING NURSING CAREERS INFORMATION, ADVICE, GUIDANCE OR COUNSELLING

Careers guidance, advice and counselling resources in the UK are patchy, and relatively few nurses access well-informed, impartial nursing careers advisory services or publications. In general, careers advice and guidance are usually provided by Senior Lecturers of particular specialities in your local School of Nursing, usually situated in your local university. Comprehensive careers counselling that gives an overview of all specialities and in-depth help to nurses with particular problems or interests is available, but it can be difficult to find out where it is available and to access it.

In order to make a rational career choice, you need *careers information,* that gives you the facts – that is, written and/or verbal information about career opportunities, including the number and types of posts available at a particular level and in a particular specialty, and details of the qualifications and training necessary. *Careers guidance* is more personal and directive, and provides advice within the context of the opportunities that are available. It is useful for those who have not made a career decision or who have decided on their career goal but are uncertain about the best way of achieving it. *Careers counselling* is a more intensive process requiring specialist skills. Ideally, careers counselling builds on careers advice or guidance, appraisal and assessment, and pastoral support. It includes the recognition and analysis of a person's strengths and weaknesses with regard to available career options.

Careers counselling involves a facilitatory approach for nurses who are uncertain of their career direction, or who have particular career problems, e.g. those who have a health disability or whose career is constrained by personal circumstances, or who appear to be unsuited to their current post.[13,14]

Established nurses who want to change their career direction may require careers information, careers guidance, careers counselling or personal counselling, depending on their individual circumstances and how far they have progressed with career planning.

Effective careers services should be 'available, accessible, appropriate, accurate, impartial, confidential, performed by people who have been trained to do it, and responsive to culture and gender,' according to the British Medical Association,[14] and this advice is also appropriate for nurses. For most nurses the type of careers advice they have received, if any, has been of the 'be like me' variety, with senior nurses describing their own careers as appropriate role models.

Nurses who are born with or develop a disability experience discrimination at work, where colleagues may be reluctant to accommodate their special needs, and there can be problems with nursing education held in venues with poor access for the disabled. The NHS cannot afford to continue to maintain such negative attitudes to disabled nurses, not only because it should be acting as a good role model for other organisations in optimising the working potential of those with disabilities, but also because of the current threat to nursing workforce numbers in many areas of the UK. Targeted help and support might increase the numbers who stay in active nursing practice for longer, whether they be nurses who have become disabled by stress and other mental health problems, or those who are physically disabled or suffering from chronic ill health.

EXERCISE 7   Do you know where you could obtain careers information, advice, guidance or counselling?

Think back – have you ever received such help? (*Yes/No*)

If so, was it from someone who was experienced, well informed and gave impartial advice, and who had dedicated time to spend with you? (*Yes/No*)

Do you know where to obtain such information, advice or counselling? Does your local higher education institution or university have generic careers advisers who you might consult, or might they advise you as to where other professional career advice is available?

The more skills you have the more marketable you will be, and the more you can dictate your pay and conditions. However, you may need assertiveness skills to make sure that others offering the post understand the skills, knowledge and experience you will be bringing to it, and to negotiate a good rate of pay. If you think that by undertaking a job you will become better known in the area or that it will subsequently attract extra work or custom, you may choose to do the initial job for little or no pay, but don't let people assume that you will do a job for free – only do so by your own choice.

Find a buddy, mentor, co-tutor or coach

You have made a good start by working through this book and reassessing your career and how satisfied you are with different aspects of it. You will be more likely to follow your action plans and overcome hiccups in your progress if you have a trusted friend or adviser with whom to discuss your career path.

You might ask a friend who is a nurse in another team or similar post, and meet regularly to listen to each other, give practical or emotional support, swap information and identify possible solutions. Someone with whom you have such an equal relationship might be described as a buddy, a co-tutor or a peer supporter.

A mentor relationship would be a more one-way relationship in which the mentor had the time and capacity to listen to you and help to facilitate your making decisions about your career. A mentor is usually a senior colleague whom the 'mentee' (the person being mentored) respects and trusts, and who has had working experience that is relevant to the mentee. Some mentors are only concerned with helping the nurse being mentored to identify and meet their educational or training needs through a development plan, whereas others are prepared to give practical or emotional support as well. A regular appraisal of your career once a year by someone who is interested and whose opinion you respect is a great way to boost your morale and motivation.

A coach could offer more directive help about your career in the same way that a sports coach urges on an athlete. Coaching involves training, supporting, instructing and motivating others to improve their performance by a working partnership between client and coach to achieve agreed goals. A good coach is said to have psychology, business and communication skills. Coaches work through one-to-one conversations either in person or by email.

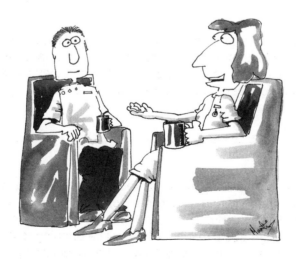

▼

'Buddies'.

EXERCISE 8   With whom could you discuss your career development?

Now that you have read some suggestions about finding someone with whom to discuss your career progress or aspirations, you should think about how that applies to you. What kind of confidant might suit you? (e.g. a nurse mentor, non-nursing careers adviser, a buddy)

Have you any particular person in mind who you might engage in such a relationship?

Write down at least three topics that you would like to discuss in this way, e.g. possibilities for career development.

And finally

EXERCISE 9   Reassess your current job by summarising the positive and negative factors relating to it and making a timetabled action plan for taking your career forward.

The positive factors will include the good aspects of your job, what makes it worthwhile, and why you do it. The negative factors will include the down-side of your job, and what you would change if you could.

Positive factors:

Negative factors:

How does the positive side compare with the negative side? (*Positive side outweighs the negative side/About equal/Negative side outweighs the positive side*)

Do you want to make changes, e.g. change your current job, change to a different way of working?

EXERCISE 9   Continued.

What are your new goals?

What actions will you take to achieve your goals, e.g. gain new skills, look at advertisements, undertake personality assessment, etc.? Who can help? When?

-

-

-

-

When will you review your progress with your career development?

References

1 Institute for Employment Studies (1996) *In the balance: registered nurse supply and demand.* Royal College of Nursing, London.

2 Maslow AH (1970) *Motivation and personality.* Harper and Row, New York.

3 Wheeler H (1997) Nurse occupational stress research. 2. Definition and conceptualization. *Br J Nurs.* **6**: 710–13.

4 Holding D (1998) *Pre-registration nurse education annual monitoring report.* Staffordshire University, Stafford.

5 English National Board (1998) *Annual Report of the English National Board for Nursing, Midwifery and Health Visiting.* English National Board, London.

6 Myers Briggs I, Myers P (1996) *Gifts differing. Understanding personality type.* Davies-Black Publishing, California.

7 Schein E (1990) *Career anchors; discovering your real needs.* Pfeiffer and Company, Oxford.

8 English National Board for Nursing, Midwifery and Health Visiting (ENB) (1992) *Framework for continuing professional education and training and higher award for nurses, midwives and health visitors.* ENB, London.

9 United Kingdom Central Council for Nursing, Midwifery and Health Visiting (UKCC) (1998) *A higher level of practice consultation document.* UKCC, London.

10 United Kingdom Central Council for Nursing, Midwifery and Health Visiting (UKCC) (1997) *Framework of standards for the preparation of teachers of nursing, midwifery and health visiting.* UKCC, London.

11 Ashburner L (1997) Defining role. *Health Serv J.* **17**: 32–3.

12 Royal College of Nursing (1997) *Nurse practitioners.* Royal College of Nursing, London.

13 Royal College of Nursing (1998) *RCN directions.* Royal College of Nursing, London.

14 British Medical Association (1996) *Guidelines for the provision of careers services for doctors.* British Medical Association, London.

RESOURCES

Books and information leaflets

Alexander L (1997) *Career networking.* How to Books Ltd, Oxford.

Booher D (1997) *Get ahead, stay ahead! Learn the 70 most important career skills, traits and attitudes to stay employed, get promoted, get a better job.* McGraw-Hill, London.

Clifton D, Nelson P (1994) *Play to your strengths.* Piatkus Publishers Ltd, London.

Cormack D (ed.) (1990) *Developing your career in nursing.* Chapman & Hall, London.

Eggert M (1992) *The perfect CV: all you need to get it right first time.* Arrow Business Books, London.

Francis D (1994) *Managing your own career.* Harper Collins, London.

Handy C (1995) *The age of unreason.* Arrow Business Books, London.

Leider R (1994) *Life skills: taking charge of your personal and professional growth.* Pfeiffer and Company, London.

Myers Briggs I, Myers P (1980) *Gifts differing. Understanding personality types.* Davies-Black Publishing, California.

Nelson Bolles R (1996) *What colour is your parachute? A practical manual for job hunters and career changers.* Ten Speed Press, California.

Pemberton C, Refause J, Evans C (1998) *Managing career dilemmas.* Financial Times Management, London.

Professional Nurse (1990) *The staff nurse's survival guide.* Austen Cornish Publishers Ltd, London.

RCN Directions. Freepost Directions, Royal College of Nursing, PO Box 33, Newport, Gwent NP1 4IN. A publication on career development. Enclose cheque for £2 made payable to RCN Publishing Company.

Turner B (ed.) (1998) *The writer's handbook 1998.* Macmillan, London.

Courses: examples

Ashridge Development Programmes for Executives. Ashridge is an international centre for management and organisation development. Courses range from short day programmes in strategic management, leadership, performance and personal skills to one-year full-time or several years part-time MBA or general manager programmes. Contact: Ashridge Management College, Berkhamsted, Hertfordshire HP4 1NS. Email *info@ashridge.org.uk*

Centre for Health Planning and Management, University of Keele, runs senior management programmes, the diploma in management for doctors, nurses and other health professionals, and full-time and part-time MBA (Health Executive) programme. Contact: Darwin Building, University of Keele, Keele, Staffordshire ST5 5BG. Fax: 01782 711737.

Health Services Management Centre, University of Birmingham, runs leadership and management development programmes for senior managers and clinicians in the NHS, as well as a range of targeted short courses. Contact: Park House, 40 Edgbaston Park Road, Birmingham B15 2RT. Internet: *http://www.bham.ac.uk/hsmc/*

Health Services Management Unit, University of Manchester, runs NHS management development programmes. Contact: Devonshire House, University Precinct Centre, Oxford Road, Manchester M13 9PL. Fax: 0161 273 5245.

Institute of Health and Care Development (IHCD) runs career development programmes and undertakes consultancy on organisational development issues. It is supported by the NHS Executive and provides the officially endorsed Career Management Programmes for mid-career NHS staff in England. Contact: IHCD, St Bartholomews Court, 18 Christmas Street, Bristol BS1 5BT. Tel: 0117 929 1029. Internet: *http://www.ihcd.org.uk*

King's Fund Management College runs programmes for general management, personal and professional development and leadership aimed at improving the clinical, professional and managerial leadership of the NHS. Contact: 11–13 Cavendish Square, London W1M OAN. Tel: 0171 307 2400. Internet: *http://www.kingsfund.org.uk*

Open University Business School runs management development programmes, including MBA. The Centre for Higher Education Practice in the Open University runs the postgraduate certificate in teaching and learning in higher education and other higher education courses. Contact: The Open University, Milton Keynes MK7 6AA. Fax: 01908 858438. Internet: *http://cehep.open.ac.uk*

Organisations

Avens Consultancy provides coaching, skills training and self-development programmes. Contact: Woodcock Delph Fenny Drayton, Ashbourne, Derbyshire DE6 1LA. Telephone and fax: 01335 350540. Internet: *gharrisavens@msn.com*

Career Dilemmas Forum has set up a network to support organisations and individuals in overcoming specific career dilemmas by giving practical help.

It offers coaching and mentoring support, career counselling, skills training, career workshops and self-development support programmes. Contact: The Corn House, Tathall End, Hanslope, Buckinghamshire MK19 7NF.

Career Management Service runs a programme for NHS professionals. It offers a service for individuals who aspire to senior posts in the NHS, or who want to maximise their performance and job satisfaction in their present posts via personal development plans. Contact: Career Management, St Bartholomews Court, 18 Christmas Street, Bristol BS1 5BT. Fax: 0117 925 0574.

Career Track International supplies seminars and audio- and video-tapes on management and leadership skills, appraisal, team-building, stress management, delegation, mastering change, motivation, computing and personal skills, such as building self-esteem. Contact: Career Track International, Sunrise House, Sunrise Parkway, Linford Wood, Milton Keynes MK14 6YA. Tel: 01908 354101 (tapes); 01908 354000 (seminars). Internet: *http://www.careertrack.com*

English National Board for Nursing, Midwifery and Health Visiting. Contact: Victory House, 170 Tottenham Court Road, London WIP OHA. Tel: 0171 391 6200. NHS Careers, PO Box 376, Bristol BS99 3EY. Tel: 0845 606 0655. Fax: 0117 921 9561.

Health Service Careers publishes a number of booklets which provide information about different nursing careers. These are *HSC2 Mental Health Nursing: working in partnership, HSC3 Midwifery: meet someone new everyday, HSC4 Children's Nursing: involves the whole family, HSC7 Nursing: it makes you think* and *HSC8 Learning Disability Nursing: bringing quality to life*. Contact: PO Box 204, London SE99 7UW. Tel: 0171 636 6287.

Institute of Personnel and Development (IPD) is a European organisation that deals with the management and development of people. The publications and training packs offer educational resources in these fields. Distributors: Plymbridge Distributors Ltd, Estover, Plymouth PL6 7PZ. Internet: *http://www.ipd.co.uk*

Medical Defence Union Ltd, 192 Altrincham Road, Manchester M22 4RZ. Tel: Freephone 0800 716376. Fax: 0161 491 1420.

National Board for Nursing, Midwifery and Health Visiting in Northern Ireland has a team of professional advisers. Contact: 79 Chichester Street, Belfast BT1 4JE. Tel: 012332 2338152.

National Board for Nursing, Midwifery and Health Visiting in Scotland. Contact: Careers Information Service, 22 Queen Street, Edinburgh EH2 1NT. Tel: 0131 225 2096.

National Board for Nursing, Midwifery and Health Visiting in Wales has a careers information service which can be contacted by telephone. Contact: Second Floor, Golate House, 101 St Mary Street, Cardiff CF1 1DX. Tel: 01222 261400.

NHS Senior Career Development Service/Executive Choice is run by Dearden Management in association with the Health Services Management Unit at the University of Manchester. The service is aimed at managers and clinicians working just below Board level. It offers career counselling and coaching, training, briefing and networking. Membership includes a regular newsletter, access to master classes on personal and professional development skills and coaching. Contact: Executive Choice, Deaden Management, Church Road, Redial, Bristol BS18 7SG. Fax: 01934 863390. Internet: *http://www.nhs-ExecChoice.co.uk*

Resource Systems will assess individuals' personal profiles using an in-house Occupational Stress Indicator administered as an interactive CD-ROM with personal feedback. The report highlights level of job satisfaction, levels of drive, patience and influence, effects of pressure, sources of pressure, behavioural style and coping, and aims to give the individual insights into the way they manage pressure at work and in the rest of their lives.

Royal College of Nursing, 20 Cavendish Square, London W1M 0AB. Tel: 0171 409 3333.

United Kingdom Central Council for Nursing, Midwifery and Health Visiting (UKCC). Contact: 23 Portland Place, London WIN 4JT. Tel: 0171 637 7181. The UKCC has a professional advice service which handles enquires relating to all aspects of the UKCC's standards for practice, education and conduct. The telephone number for this service is 0171 333 6541/6550/6553.